Boy Giant

The Story Of Robert Wadlow
The World's Tallest Man

by Dan Brannan

Printed in the United States of America

First Edition – October 2003

ISBN 0-9650228-5-4

Published by Alton Museum of History and Art
2809 College Ave.
Alton, IL 62002

Printed by Faith Printing Co.
4210 Locust Hill Road
Taylors, SC 29687

Table of Contents

Foreword   *iv*
Dedication   *vi*
Author Biography   *vii*

Chapter 1   — A Giant Kindergartener   *1*
Chapter 2   — Child Grows Into Giant   *6*
Chapter 3   — The Tallest Scout   *12*
Chapter 4   — Just A Growing Boy   *18*
Chapter 5   — Land Of Giants   *25*
Chapter 6   — College Bound   *31*
Chapter 7   — A Devoted Christian   *41*
Chapter 8   — Travels In The Big Apple   *46*
Chapter 9   — A Doctor's Betrayal; Westward Travels   *54*
Chapter 10 — Coming To Trial   *62*

Photo Section   *69*

Chapter 11 — Seeing The U.S.A   *93*
Chapter 12 — Death Of A Giant   *102*
Chapter 13 — The Funeral Of Robert Wadlow   *109*
Chapter 14 — A Photographer's Favorite Subject   *114*
Chapter 15 — Preserving The Wadlow Legend   *119*
Chapter 16 — The Wadlow Statue   *123*
Chapter 17 — Wadlow, An International Sensation   *130*
Chapter 18 — Wadlow, Medical Analysis   *136*
Chapter 19 — Alton's Favorite Son   *142*
Chapter 20 — Family Reunion   *147*

Alton, Illinois Key Historical Facts   *155*
Boy Giant Order Form   *157*
Life to The Fullest Order Form   *158*

Boy Giant

Foreword

My father, Bob Brannan, was a blue-eyed, brown-haired boy clinging to his mother's hand in Snyders Department Store on Third Street in Alton, Ill., in 1936, when he looked up and saw the most astonishing sight of his life — 18-year-old Robert Wadlow, who stood more than 8 feet tall and weighed close to 400 pounds.

Robert Wadlow was grasping the hand of his baby brother, Harold Jr. My father said that when he saw Robert, it was as if everyone in the store was frozen, with eyes focused on Robert. Robert proceeded as if everything was normal and went about his business of looking at clothing items.

"There he is, there is the tallest man in the world," my dad's mother said in a hushed tone.

That night, my father, grandmother, Julia, and grandfather, Charles, talked about the day's big event of seeing Robert Wadlow. That conversation is still a cherished Brannan family memory.

My father, Bob, died in February 2002 after a brave battle with colon/liver cancer. My dad was my most ardent supporter.

When I moved to Alton in May 1997, our home was directly across the street from where the Wadlow family had lived. It must have been fate that I would eventually write the definitive Wadlow biography. During our time there, I would sometimes sneak a glimpse down the street and imagine what the neighborhood must have been like some 60 years earlier when Robert was carrying his 8-foot frame down the street hand in hand with Harold Jr.

I hope this book provides a glimpse at Robert Wadlow that only his brother, Harold Jr., and close friends have carried since his death. Most of those memories are in this book.

Dedication

The image of bright-eyed toddler Harold Wadlow Jr. peeking around his 8-foot-8-inch brother, Robert, is a cherished memory embedded in Alton, Ill., history. Leland Heppner's 1939 Boy Giant cover photo at the family home on Sanford Avenue in Alton captures the essence of their relationship.

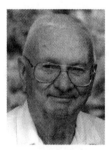

Harold Wadlow Jr.
1932-2000

Harold Wadlow Jr. died unexpectedly during the writing of this book at 5:19 p.m. Dec. 31, 2000, at Alton Memorial Hospital. I dedicate this book to him.

Thanks to Charlene Gill, Vickie Kinney, Steve Whitworth, Charlotte Stetson, Phil Gonzales, Debbie Shouse and Vicki Bennington for their editing input. Also thanks to Georgia Mills for the cover and back cover design and Robert Graul, John Badman and the late Heppner for the photography in the book.

I also dedicate the book to my two girls, Savannah and Sierra, and my devoted wife, Victoria. Since the day I met her, Victoria has been the light of my life. I hope the book will help Savannah and Sierra take to future generations Robert's message that despite physical obstacles and incessant public attention, one can remain kind and gentle to others.

About the Author

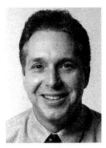

Dan Brannan has been in journalism since 1978 at Eastern Illinois University in Charleston, Ill. He started his professional career in 1982 as a sports writer at the Daily Union in Shelbyville, Ill. He is the executive editor of The Telegraph in Alton, Ill., a 30,000 circulation daily newspaper.

Brannan has been at The Telegraph since 1997 and has led the newspaper to more than 100 awards during his tenure, including four General Excellence awards in Illinois Press Association, Southern Illinois Editorial Association and Journal Register Company contests. In 2001, The Telegraph placed first in the IPA General Excellence competition and second in 2002. The Telegraph was first in the Southern Illinois contest in 2002. The Telegraph was first in the 1999 Journal Register Company front page contest for design and content.

Brannan's newspaper in Seneca/Clemson, S.C., also placed first in General Excellence in 1995 and third in 1996.

After his start in sports in the early 1980s, Brannan was promoted to managing editor at age 27 in 1988 at a publication in Sikeston, Mo. The Sikeston newspaper had the highest circulation increase in the United States for all newspapers in 1989. Brannan was hired as managing editor of a newspaper double in circulation size in Rocky Mount, N.C., and led the newspaper to historic circulation highs and earned national and international prominence in the Thomson newspaper company from 1990 to the mid-1990s. In the early 1990s, The Telegram in Rocky Mount earned first place in investigative reporting, the most prestigious category in the state.

Brannan has written three other books: "The Courage To Live," a biography about Donna Gustavel, a young woman with multiple disabilities in February 1997; "Everyday Angels," an inspirational book of moving human interest stories, published in 1996; and "Life To The Fullest: Stories Of People Coping With Diabetes," approved by the National American Diabetes Association in 1995.

Boy Giant

Chapter 1

A Giant Kindergartener

Robert Wadlow bravely climbed the stairs into Roxana Elementary School in Roxana, Ill., for the first day of kindergarten.

Robert was a typical 5-year-old boy, with a curious, intelligent nature. He had thin, blond hair and ocean-blue eyes. The only thing that wasn't typical about Robert was his size. He stood 5-feet-4 and weighed 105 pounds as he entered kindergarten.

There had been talk around Roxana of Robert's first day in school for several months as word spread through the neighborhood of his incredible height. Students and teachers alike seemed to freeze as Robert strolled hand in hand with his mother and father into school halls for the first time.

Robert's mother, Addie, and father, Harold, squeezed each of Robert's hands as he made his journey into the classroom. Addie was slim, with dark hair, and more withdrawn than the outgoing Harold. Harold was of medium height and slim build. Harold was the talker in the Wadlow family and always had something to say to friend or stranger.

That day in 1923 was typical of the fall; muggy and humid in the Mississippi River town. The air seemed to hang, and the temperatures inside the Roxana school hovered near the century mark. Robert started school at 5 1/2 years old in September 1923 and was already wearing a suit for a boy of 17 years old.

As Robert walked down the hall toward his kindergarten class, some of the teachers started to step outside their classrooms to see the young giant. "There he is, the little giant," one teacher whispered to another.

When Robert, Harold and Addie entered the room, all the kids gazed in amazement. Robert towered over the rest of them, standing as tall as many 13- and 14-year-olds.

Robert slipped into a seat with his name on it. It was not an easy fit. He had to force his large body into the miniature seat made for kindergarteners.

Robert was a normal-sized boy when he was born Feb. 22, 1918, in a small five-room cottage on Monroe Street in Alton. The attending physician reported that Robert's weight of 8 1/2 pounds and length were normal for a baby boy, but nothing else in life would ever be normal for Robert. Robert's exact length at birth was never recorded.

The United States had been engulfed in World War I a few years earlier, and it was clear America, a previously sleeping giant, was awakening into a rich, booming, international power. America had gone from a rural, agricultural base to a country with strong industrial production. Alton/Roxana, Ill., was a vibrant part of that industrial process, with oil refineries and factories and access to the nearby Mississippi River. Roxana was built around the Shell Refinery, one of the area's largest employers. Alton was also a steamboat town, with many steamers visiting the river city on journeys up and down the Mississippi.

Robert Pershing Wadlow was named for John Joseph Pershing, commander in chief of U.S. forces during World War I. Pershing was originally from Marceline, Mo., and was a well-known hero in the St. Louis area. Pershing's recognition throughout the St. Louis region influenced the Wadlows' choice of a middle name for their son Robert.

Harold Wadlow was employed by a construction company at an oil refinery in Wood River, Ill., at the time of Robert's birth. Shortly after Robert's birth, Harold decided to transfer to Charleston, West Virginia, hoping to improve the family's financial fortunes.

The Wadlow family stayed in West Virginia for a short period of time, then returned to the Alton area, moving to Grafton, a village about 20 miles from Alton at the confluence of the Illinois and Mississippi rivers, before settling in Roxana. Robert continued to grow and grow and at 6 months weighed 30 pounds. At one year, he weighed 45 pounds, and at 1 1/2 years he weighed 67 pounds. There were no medical records of Robert's height during those first 18 months.

Harold and Addie were startled and worried about Robert's extraordinary growth. At that time, not much was known about Robert's overactive pituitary gland. In the fall of the following year, doctors diagnosed Robert with a double hernia. A 3-hour operation was performed at St. Joseph's Hospital in Alton. He was hospitalized for 17 days and recovered without incident. Robert's first three siblings were born two years apart, Helen in 1920; Eugene H. in 1922; and Betty Jean in 1924. All were of a normal length and weight when they were born.

Robert's teachers considered him a highly intelligent child, who had no problem learning the different kindergarten tasks. The social side of school was not always easy for Robert during his first year. It seemed that the kids were always staring at him, and teachers spent an equal amount of time gawking. In games of hide-and-go-seek, Robert was usually not successful because he always towered over the bushes and any type of cover.

Sometimes the kids allowed themselves to be found so Robert wouldn't be "it" all the time. Robert was almost always "it" during games of hide-and-go-seek.

Addie walked Robert to school each day, watching over her young son. Harold had to go to his job, so he couldn't walk with them, but when Harold wasn't working, he spent time with Robert, and they had a strong bond. The Wadlows knew that soon Robert would need a larger chair and table at school, because he didn't fit any of those in the kindergarten class.

At lunch time each day, Addie went to the school to retrieve her son. Robert welcomed her with open arms, running in clumsy fashion to greet her. He was enjoying the schooling, but he loved being home with his mother. After school, Robert and his mother often went to the supermarket or a city park. Usually several people followed them, watching their every move. Robert was already an attraction around the area for youngsters and adults alike. It was only to be the beginning of an endless stream of public curiosity.

By age 8, Robert had grown to an even 6 feet and weighed 169 pounds. Robert got his first mention in the Alton Telegraph in March 1926 with the headline, "Here's Robert Wadlow and His Size 17 Shoes."

The shoes were made to order through Tom and Bob's Boot Shop in Alton. Robert's foot had already outgrown the measuring stick at the shop, and a tape line had to be used in determining the shoe size when the order was given to the Bloomer shoe factory. The shoes were 19 inches long. At 8 years old, Robert had the appearance of a youth of 19 or 20 years and was considered the largest boy in the world for his age. Robert's socks cost 75 cents a pair, compared to the average of three pairs for a dollar. A new pair of shoes cost him $30.

The Wadlows moved from Roxana to Alton, and Robert transferred to Milton School. By the time he was a pupil in the fifth grade, he was 6 feet 2 1/2 inches tall and weighed 195 pounds.

During that period he appeared in a movie newsreel filmed by a St. Louis representative of Pathe News showing his phenomenal height. The Pathe News representative visited Milton

School during the noon hour and took seven views of Robert. Later, the newsreel photographer went to the Wadlow home and filmed Robert with his father. Wadlow's photo also appeared in the St. Louis Globe-Democrat at that time. He was 2 1/2 inches taller than his father and weighed 75 pounds more than his mother.

When Robert was 8 years old, a bus driver tried to make him pay adult fare. Robert's father, Harold Sr., challenged the bus driver and said, "But he's only in the third grade."

"Prove it," the conductor said.

Harold Sr. pondered for a moment and said, "Okay, drive us three blocks out of your way to our home and I'll get you his birth certificate." The driver rejected the offer and told them to go ahead and sit down on the bus. Robert later experienced the same problem with a conductor when he tried to board a train.

"Ten bucks says he's only eight," Harold Wadlow Sr. told the conductor. The rail conductor then backed down and Robert rode for free.

Ruth Minard met Robert for the first time at Milton School when Robert was 9. She went to Milton School then to Alton High School with him. It wasn't Robert's height that impressed Minard but his heartwarming smile. As she walked to Milton School each day with him she felt he was "a ray of sunshine." "He lit up the whole block when he walked," Minard said. "You could just feel his love for other people."

Robert would carry that love and compassion of people through the remainder of his life.

Chapter 2

Child Grows Into Giant

S.W. Harris, St. Louis chapter president of the National Society of Long Fellows, had heard tales of the boy giant from Alton and decided to make a trip in person to extend a personal invitation to the 6-foot-4-inch school boy to join the club. The minimum height requirements for membership was 6-feet-1 in shoes. The society was formed in 1927 in Topeka, Kan., and then had 1,500 members.

"Hi, Robert," Harris said when he was introduced to Robert and his family at their home.

Harris happened to have a tape measure with him and asked his father to take the tape and stretch it out. "Robert, can you take off your shoes?" Harris asked. Robert said, "Sure, Mr. Harris."

Robert stepped up the tape and topped the 6-foot-4 mark with Harris' tape measure. Harris' eyes almost popped out of their sockets. "You are for real, aren't you young man?" he asked.

"Well, sir, I guess I am," Robert said politely.

By age 10, Robert was 6-foot-5 and 210 pounds. Doctors estimated at that point that Robert would be at least 8 feet tall when he finished growing. Robert's father was 5-foot-8, 140 pounds, and Robert could easily lift his father off the floor. In early 1928, the regular desks at Milton School were too small for Robert. School officials transferred a seat from the high school and added 6-inch blocks to make it tall enough for him.

The new seat was high enough but not strong enough and broke down. Next an armchair was provided. Robert's chair was always in the back of the room, otherwise the other children could not see the teacher or the blackboard over him. The desk wasn't the typical chair kind of desk. The desk was in front, and he normally slid down into the seat.

Robert also had problems getting in and out of the family Ford sedan even during his grade school days. Robert had little leg room in the rear seat, and his head just missed the top of the car by a half inch.

The first time Henry B. Lenhardt saw Robert, Robert's father was driving a two-door Ford down a hill on Humbert Street in Alton next to a small parking lot. When Robert's father parked the car, it seemed to take Robert forever to unwind himself out of the back seat.

Alton's Harold Swinney first met Robert Wadlow in May 1928, living just a "high weed patch" away from Robert. The pair became instant friends, following an ice wagon for a piece of ice. One of the pair's first projects together was to build a hut from the high weeds near their respective homes. "We patterned the hut after one built by the natives of foreign lands as it appeared in our geography books," recalled Swinney.

Robert and Swinney walked together to Horace Mann School in the morning, went home at noon for lunch, walked back to school together and home again at 3:30 p.m. Then the two changed clothes and played together until suppertime. Sometimes the inseparable pair had snacks in their weed hut.

Robert and Swinney often played marbles on the cindered drive. Like most boys playing marbles, sometimes they did not agree. Swinney's mother could see the two children playing from her back door. Swinney's mother told friends: "I was in the kitchen and looked out to see Bob and Harold playing marbles. When I looked out again, Bob and Harold were fighting. Some people asked her, 'What did you do?' She would reply, 'Nothing. I just went on preparing supper. When I looked out again, Bob and Harold were playing marbles again. Bob was good-natured, but boys will be boys, and Bob was a boy.'"

Swinney and Robert each had B.B. guns; Daisy single shots. Living near the railroad tracks, Harold and Robert walked a wellknown path between the railroad tracks and their homes and used the B.B. guns to shoot cans for target practice.

On Saturdays, Robert and Swinney would pull their coaster wagons and convince neighbors to hire them to haul off their tin cans and bottles. The boys had an area near their homes where no one objected to the pair dumping cans. Afterward Robert and Swinney took the dime apiece that they earned and walked to Upper Alton to see a serial movie usually of a Western nature starring Hoot Gibson, Tom Mix or Buck Jones. When weather permitted, the two used to walk down to Wood River Creek and cross the C & A Railroad Bridge. "It took us 15 or 20 minutes to get to the bend of the creek," Swinney said. "There we would go swimming."

Swinney and Robert Wadlow attended summer school together at Milton School and also at Horace Mann. The two walked to Milton in the morning and to Horace Mann after going home for lunch. Both learned a lot, and quickly learned that if their attendance was good, they were given a free ticket to go swimming at the Lindbergh Swimming Pool on Friday afternoon.

Children at the pool named for Charles A. Lindbergh, the first man to cross the Atlantic Ocean in a single-engine plane, could often be heard chanting: "Here comes Robbie, expect the water to come up!" Robert would be up to his ears in water in a matter of seconds before he realized kids were shouting at him.

In the fall of 1928, Robert was 6 feet 11 inches tall, a gain of an inch in five months, and weighed 248 pounds, also a slight gain. He had been measured for a new pair of shoes, size 27 — two sizes larger than his last pair. They were to be manufactured by the Bloomer Shoe Co. for the Tom & Bob Shop at the former's factory in Racine, Wis., and cost $50.

Dorothy Carter Hagen was a close neighbor of the Wadlows. One Christmas, Dorothy and Robert each received a shiny red sled. The Hagens had a hill in their yard, just right for sleigh riding. "Bob let us know that he got a Flexible Flyer and would come down as soon as it snowed," Hagen said. "Back then our home was at a dead-end street, no traffic... no fences... just right for children with new sleds. In a few days it snowed, and we children would have chores to do before we could go out and try the hill. Mrs. Wadlow and Mama would talk about what we should wear then they set a time limit on the time we could stay out. Robert lived a block away and often came to play at our house, then we would go inside for some home-made cookies."

Hagen's mother used to caution Robert about being careful when he walked up and down the steps of their porch because his feet were so big. Robert didn't know it at the time, but Hagen's father secretly watched the boards when he stepped on their porch to make sure they were strong enough to support him. Once Hagen's father asked Robert what he ate for breakfast, and he bluntly responded, "Just everything my mother puts out."

Sophia Davis studied with Robert at Milton School. Once, Davis was stunned to see the unusual sight of Robert jumping up and down in class with the other boys nearly half his size. Mr. Zeiler, the teacher, was passing out some treats, and the boys were jumping around to get his attention, even though Robert was much taller than Zeiler. "Mr. Zeiler, Mr. Zeiler, I want a treat," Robert hollered. Mr. Zeiler rapidly rewarded that tall boy with a treat.

Leland Duncan met Robert Wadlow in the summer of 1928. Duncan's parents had recently moved from North Alton to Dorothy Street in Upper Alton. Looking across Brown Street and toward Milton Road, Duncan saw a man (he thought) scooting along in a small coaster wagon. He froze, staring at the moving giant.

"All kids used to put one knee in the wagon bed and used the other leg and foot to propel the wagon along," Duncan said. "The thing I remember the most was about 18 inches of leg hanging out the back of the wagon bed and this big foot dragging down along the sidewalk. There were a couple of other kids playing with Robert, and when he got up from the wagon, I could hardly believe what I was seeing. He was as big as my dad and only 10 years old at that time. I had never heard of him or seen him before."

Walter Bratten used to play with Robert when Robert was 9 or 10 years old on Brown Street in Alton when he visited his grandmother, Molly Morgan. "Robert never got to first base when we played baseball because he had trouble running, but he could hit the ball," Bratten said. "We used to play cops and robbers and we used to shoot cap guns together."

Harold Shipley moved to an Alton home just off Brown Street, across from the Wadlows, in 1928. One of Shipley's favorite activities with Robert was playing tag.

"I was always the runner, he was the catcher," Shipley said. "I was small for my age; my mother was always afraid Robert would step on me. His shoes were almost as long as I was tall. Needless to say, this never happened. He was six years older and four times taller than me."

Tom Weber also met Robert in 1928. He lived in the 3300 block of Brown Street in Alton, while Wadlow lived in the 3200 block. Weber played the groom in a Tom Thumb Wedding staged for second and third graders at Milton School. Robert

Wadlow, a fourth grader, played the minister, and Genevieve Wilson played the bride. Weber and Wilson were both 8 years old at the time and in the second grade at Milton School.

It was not uncommon to find Robert Wadlow in any Milton School play. Robert added celebrity status and any time he was involved in an Alton public event, a crowd was guaranteed.

Weber wore a black tuxedo for the Tom Thumb Wedding, while Wilson had a special dress with flowers around the top in her veil. Weber's head only reached Robert's shoulder during the Parent Teachers Association event, which drew a capacity classroom crowd.

"It was a special moment in my life," she said. "Robert ripped his trousers before the Tom Thumb Wedding started and had to run home and change them. He sure wore big trousers."

Robert remained calm during the whole wedding, never letting anyone or performing in front of an audience unnerve him. When Robert declared to Weber and Wilson: "I now pronounce you man and wife," everyone — students, faculty and parents — erupted in a thunderous applause. The Tom Thumb pastor appearance would be the first of many in the public spotlight for Robert in a life that would achieve great fame.

Chapter 3

The Tallest Scout

On Oct. 24, 1929, Robert Wadlow's life changed, as did everyone else's in America. It was Black Thursday, the day the New York Stock Exchange crashed, ending the "Roaring Twenties" and beginning the Great Depression. By the end of the day, the stock market had lost $4 billion. On Monday, Oct. 28, 1929, a full panic ensued and thousands of investors were financially ruined. At the close of the year in 1929, stock values had fallen by $15 billion.

As 1930 began, banks throughout the country and greater Alton area couldn't continue to operate. Many area farmers fell into bankruptcy. Hundreds of area families struggled to make ends meet.

Soon after the stock market crash, people lined up for sacks of free government surplus food. The Salvation Army in Alton opened daily to feed a line of destitute residents. The Alton area was fortunate to have Shell Oil, Western Cartridge Co., Standard Oil, Laclede Steel and Owens-Illinois providing jobs for some residents, but the economy remained difficult. The major employers in the region couldn't maintain their previous work force.

Residents were forced to heat their homes with wood stoves because coal was no longer available for the masses. Alton families often stood by the local railroad tracks waiting for big chunks of coal to be thrown off by the train motion.

Civilian Conservation Corps camps also began to open around the area, employing many young men. Most simply didn't have money available for shoes, clothes or food, and the CCC camps provided work erecting buildings and sidewalks.

At age 13, Robert Wadlow entered the 1930s an astonishing 7 feet tall. By Feb. 19, 1931, Robert had stretched to 7 feet 4 inches tall and weighed 282 pounds. Robert had become an attraction. Sometimes his height was a way of making a few coins for his family with personal appearances.

Robert loved typical teenage activities, including reading. He read about 300 books every year. "I like boys' adventure stories. They're sure thrilling," he once told a reporter.

Doorways became an obstacle for young Robert. Wayne Wegwart lived next door to Robert on Brown Street in Alton for about six months in the early '30s and said Robert was already bumping his head on doorways as a youngster.

"He had to stoop to get through doorways, even at age 12 or 13," Wegwart said.

As a 13-year-old, Robert liked mechanical things involving motors and airplanes. "I'd like to drive a car, but I can't get under the wheel," he said. "Sometimes Dad lets me steer from the back seat."

Robert was constantly ducking. One time in St. Louis, he was riding an escalator and was nearly leveled. He forgot to duck under a sign hanging above the escalator and got smacked in the head, resulting in an awful bump. "It nearly knocked me out, I guess," Robert said. "I like to ride the elevator. I normally don't even have to think about it any more. I'm usually pretty good at avoiding things. "

When Robert Wadlow walked down the street, cars stopped, and if they didn't pull over, they slowed up and people stared.

When he walked into an Alton store, everyone stopped and ogled. If he left Alton for a trip to St. Louis or another neighboring city, the staring got worse. Most Altonians were used to him and tried to not make their curiosity seem obvious.

"I'm getting used to people who follow me, too," Robert said at the time. "I just laugh at the people who look at me."

As a teen-ager, Robert Wadlow enjoyed the company of many young friends. Unfortunately, occasionally Robert was clumsy around his mates.

"Sometimes I might hit one of the boys I play with," he said. "They're always getting under my feet. I guess they forget I am so big."

Robert's love of typical teenager activities led to him officially join the Boy Scouts. Old troop records show that Robert was 7 feet 4, 272 pounds when he took the tenderfoot tests in Troop 1 at College Avenue Presbyterian Church on March 24, 1931. Robert officially joined the Scouts on April 14, 1931.

During the beginning ceremony at College Avenue Presbyterian Church, Robert Wadlow recited the Scout oath and laws, repeated the oath of allegiance to the flag and had to know how the flag was supposed to be held. He also had to tie the nine knots that are necessary for tenderfoot rank. One of the first accomplishments Robert had in Scouting was obtaining his membership.

The tenderfoot pin was the only article Wadlow wore in Scouting that was not an unusual size. The pin is in the shape of a fleur de lis, taken from the symbol of the mariner's compass. The fleur de lis and compass always point to the north. Robert Baden-Powell, the founder of Scouting, made the fleur de lis the symbol of Scouting in August 1907 when he established the organization.

On May 16, 1931, the biggest and smallest Boy Scouts in the world met in Alton. Robert and tiny Charlie Marchioli entertained visitors in a Scout demonstration at the L.J. Hartmann clothing store on West Third Street in Alton. He was a member of the Catholic Children's Home troop in Alton. Marchioli was 14 years old, only 47 inches tall and weighed 54 pounds; Robert was 13 years old, 7 feet 6 inches tall and weighed 290 pounds.

Robert Wadlow wore size 25 shoes when he entered Scouting and his neckties had to have 6 or 8 inches added so they would be long enough to tuck in at the top of the uniform vest.

Robert had to have a special Scout uniform made. It was supplied through the cooperation of the Louis J. Hartmann clothing firm, an official Scout outfitter in Alton, and a manufacturer. The factory had a special cylinder made to knit a stocking large enough for his size 16 foot. His uniform went on display at Hartmann's on May 20, 1931. The uniform was 10 to 12 feet in length and 1 1/2 feet to 2 feet wide.

Robert's name also appeared in the 1932 area Boy Scout charter, but he did not advance beyond the tenderfoot rank, according to Troop 1 historical records. Robert's name did not appear on the 1933 Scout charter.

When a Scout enters as a tenderfoot, he must know the Scout oath and law and have knowledge of the significance of the Scout badges and what they mean. For any young boy in Wadlow's time, achieving the rank of tenderfoot was relatively easy. After tenderfoot, comes the second-class badge. Back in Robert's day, a second-class badge was issued after about a month in Scouting.

The second-class badge was based on duty to God, country, others and self back in the early 1930s. A second-class rank was also based on basic first aid knowledge and passing 16 required tests. Some of the first aid items included knowledge of how to treat a cut finger, a black eye, sun burn and how to use a hand-kerchief.

Scouting was one of the passions in Robert's young life, as was reading. Robert liked doing things normal kids did as much as his size permitted. He was determined to be a Scout despite his enormous size, and he was successful at the beginning.

Scouting became more difficult for Robert because of his

physical size. Everything in Scouting and life in general is geared toward normal-sized people. But Robert's hands literally dwarfed a regular-sized mess kit. Robert's troop meetings even were held in a gymnasium so his head wouldn't hit the ceiling. He had to duck for the gymnasium door, but he could stand erect after he got into the gymnasium because the ceiling was 25 to 30 feet.

Boy Scout camping trips were a unique experience for Robert. When the Scouts went camping in those days, wall tents were used. The wall tents were made of a heavy dark bluish green water-proof material. They resembled a cabin with a peaked roof and hanging canvas.

Two tents had to be put end to end for Robert so he could sleep. He had to rest on two cots wired together. Edward Fischer camped with Robert at one of the annual jamborees on the Alton riverfront. "When Robert camped with us, it was necessary for him to sleep on two beds," Fischer said. "His shoulders on one cot and his legs stretched out on the other one."

Louis Eugene Grosh was the Scoutmaster of Robert's troop. Grosh stood only 5-foot-3, so Robert overwhelmed him in photographs. One of the most publicized Scout photos show Grosh and Robert Wadlow standing together while building lean-tos over a weekend at Riverfront Park at a Boy Scout Jamboree.

On that weekend, Mary Alma Keirle recalled the boys building the lean-tos out of straw, tree branches and whatever else they could find. The lean-to had a roof and three sides and the fourth side remained open. The Scouts placed bed rolls in the lean-tos to sleep on, and each boy cooked outside.

"I was a youngster, but I remember it was a big affair when they had the encampment Robert was involved in on the river front," she said. "Many people came to see the encampment."

One might think Alton people treated Robert differently while he was in Scouting, but Keirle said he was embraced as if he was just like other kids. Alton residents gave Robert his space during his time in Scouting and didn't overwhelm him by seeking autographs or posing for photographs.

Being a child celebrity because of his size wasn't easy for young Robert. At first, the Wadlow family didn't realize that Robert was a celebrity. The public didn't realize he was 13 years old and a child like other 13-year-olds, but just a lot bigger. At 13, Robert was bigger than all the grown men around. Robert would never have any privacy the rest of his life.

An Alton Evening Telegraph headline on Oct. 15, 1931, reported a Wadlow mishap: "Robert Wadlow Nursing Injured Foot in Hospital. Infection Follows Bruise Suffered While Swimming." "Robert Wadlow, Alton's Big Boy, who has attained a national prominence because of his great size, is still at Barnes Hospital Tuesday evening. He is suffering from an infection of one of his feet, which resulted from a bruise received several weeks ago while in a swimming pool. The bruise failed to clear up and a week ago, he began complaining of the injured member. Alarming symptoms prompted a surgeon to take him to the St. Louis hospital."

A story on Oct. 21, 1931, in The Telegraph reported an update on Wadlow's recovery. The story said: "An infection that for a time threatened to result disastrously has apparently been warded off, and Robert Wadlow is making rapid strides toward recovery in Barnes Hospital, St. Louis, where he was taken a week ago yesterday. The infection was located in his left foot and resulted from a bruise received several weeks ago while swimming. Since he has been at the hospital, Wadlow has received mail from Italy and South America. The mail from South America was a letter written by a postal clerk Sept. 16 and received here Oct. 16."

Robert Wadlow was never one to give up easily. Unfortunately, this Barnes Hospital trip would not be his last to the medical center as he continued to sprout into uncharted heights for his age.

Chapter 4

Just A Growing Boy

Robert Wadlow's life changed forever May 12, 1932, with the birth of his brother, Harold Jr. The baby weighed 7 3/4 pounds, was of normal length and was the fifth child of Harold Sr. and Addie Wadlow. A closeness that few brothers and sisters share existed between Robert and Harold Jr. from the beginning.

Robert described Harold Jr. at the time as "a good baby and doesn't require much care." It was not uncommon to see Harold Jr. wrapped comfortably in Robert's large arms at the family home at 3204 Brown St. in Alton.

Robert didn't want the youngest Wadlow to inherit his size characteristics. "I don't want my little brother to be as big as I am; he'll have more fun if he isn't."

Robert graduated from junior high in mid-June 1932. He was 7 feet 5 inches and weighed 301 pounds. He was considered the biggest schoolboy in Alton and possibly the world when he received his certificate as an East Junior High School graduate.

One of Harold Jr.'s earliest memories was when Robert had a lemonade and soda stand in front of their Brown Street home. The stand was an easy way for Robert to bring in a few dollars for spending money during these tight financial times.

The lemonade/soda stand was set up on a card table. Robert often sat behind the table on a folding chair while Addie Wadlow was always busy inside making the lemonade. "I remember people stopping by in the front yard," Harold Jr. said. "Robert didn't do the lemonade stand too long. People were always after him to stand up. He let me drink his lemonade, but I didn't really help. I imagine my mother made all the lemonade and did all the work. A lot of them just stopped by because they wanted to know how tall he was."

Harold Jr. felt Robert's kindness and love toward him from the very beginning. "I was Robert's baby brother, and he loved me. He didn't want me to turn out like him. He wanted me to be normal size and have a normal life. He loved me better than any big brother could love me."

Tom Weber was one of Wadlow's assistants at Wadlow's lemonade/soda stand in the early 1930s. He observed Robert sitting in a large wooden chair on hot summer nights. People from surrounding towns visited Robert's lemonade stand for a look at his size.

"I remember Robert saying, 'If you buy a soda, I'll stand up.' When they would spring for a soda or two, his brother, Ed, and I would take people a soda, but he wouldn't stand up until they paid for a soda."

Leo Schmidt once stopped at Robert's lemonade stand with his boss to buy a Coke. When Robert handed the two a Coke, they noticed how the whole bottle disappeared in Robert's hand.

When Robert Wadlow turned 14, his shoe size had grown to size 34 and had to be special ordered at a cost of $86. Before the shoes could be made, a plaster cast had to be made of his foot. A last made of a special procured wood served as a pattern to make Robert's enormous shoes. Shoes of Robert's size couldn't be made from small pieces of leather. The shoes wore well and normally lasted a year.

Growing up in the home of Harold Sr. and Addie Wadlow was not always easy. Everyone seemed endlessly curious about Robert, the family's oldest child.

Harold Jr. and his sister Betty were close to Robert. "We weren't jealous of Robert," Harold Jr. said. "My sister Helen and brother Eugene were somewhat jealous," he said. "There were two years difference between Robert, Helen, Eugene, and Betty and eight years between me and Betty.

"Betty and I had the same temperament as Robert. We were mild mannered. I think Eugene and Helen sometimes felt left out."

Addie Wadlow was a quiet, gentle person. "She was like my sister Betty and I in that respect," Harold Jr. said. "Dad was a little more aggressive, but pretty kind. Dad was a good father. He was the more outgoing of the two."

Addie didn't understand a lot of the changes that were going on in the country in the early 1920s. She appreciated gaining the right to vote in 1920, but she didn't understand the Equal Rights Amendment. Addie believed a woman's place was in the home, quietly raising children and tending to their needs.

On Feb. 22, 1933, Robert turned 15 and had grown to 7 feet 8 inches and weighed 340 pounds. During the previous year, Robert had gained 3 inches in height and 39 pounds.

Later in 1933, Robert had an interesting experience picking cherries. His extraordinary size was an asset when it came to picking cherries. Robert demonstrated his cherry picking ability when he accompanied his father to the Lurton Stites fruit farm on Curvey Street in Alton. Instead of using a ladder, Robert just stood on the ground, picking cherries as high as he could reach, then pulling the limbs down. He put on a demonstration of cherry picking that not only delighted all others there, but caused Stites to laugh and say Robert "showed up" the entire cherry picking crew.

In early July 1933, Robert, 42 boys, and six Y.M.C.A. leaders went to the World's Fair in Chicago. Robert was 7 feet 8 1/2 inches tall.

James Cannon was one of those on the trip. He watched as hundreds of people stopped to stare at Robert.

"We were exposed to a lot of strangers on the World's Fair grounds," he said. "I remember one person at the World's Fair thinking Robert was on stilts. The lady pulled up his pant leg and yelled, 'He's real! He's real!' Someone then asked the lady how she'd feel if he did that to her. Robert was very interested in everything when we went to the World's Fair. It was an exciting thing."

Henry Lenhardt played basketball in gym class with Robert. Robert struggled on the hardwoods because of his size and clumsiness. The boys attended gym class twice a week. After exercising either outside or inside, gym participants had to shower and go back to a regular class. "Of course, Robert had a big problem with this, as he never moved that fast," Lenhardt said.

Lenhardt said Robert's height worked as much to his favor as it did against him if he stood under the basket. "He had the advantage — that he could be the "dropper" — he'd stand alongside the basket, someone would pass him the basketball and he'd drop it in," Lenhardt said.

Lee Duncan observed Robert as a freshman at Alton High. Robert caught Duncan's attention taking the school's stairs, as his foot was twice as long as the stair tread was deep, so he was forced to go up almost sideways.

"His feet were so huge by then that when he went up the steps he did so one step at a time with the foot sideways parallel to the step riser," Duncan said. "Of course he had a good grip on the banister all the time. When he was coming down a flight of steps, he would place his heel against the step riser letting most of the foot hang over the step. He would hang onto the banister and come down one step at a time. I assume he did this to keep his weight centered more or less in a straight line."

Most boys growing up in Upper Alton hung around the busi-

21

ness district called Pie Town, called that because, during the war with Mexico in 1846, Upper Alton ladies baked pies for soldiers from Illinois regiments camped in Alton. The name stuck through the years.

Duncan saw Robert get off a city bus numerous times at the southeast corner of an intersection in Upper Alton. "Robert always rode in the front seat next to the bus door," he said. "After the bus stopped and the door opened, the first thing one would see was two huge feet swing down to the sidewalk. Then Robert would hunch his head down and bend over as much as he could to clear the doorway. Once clear, he would stand up and his head was above the top of the bus."

Harold Swinney frequently observed Robert riding to Alton Junior High School and Alton High School with Herman Doerr in Herman's father's 1925 Model T Ford pickup truck. "The end gate was down and his long legs could be there, though his feet hung over. It was much more comfortable than squeezing into an automobile. I rode behind them on a bicycle or motor-cycle so the people in cars behind them would not get too close."

Millie Bentley, a volunteer at the Alton Museum of History & Art, saw Robert Wadlow in the early 1930s in Cape Girardeau, Mo. Robert, who was making appearances through-out the region, was the featured attraction at the department store grand opening. He handed out books of matches for men and powder puffs for women.

Bentley remembers overhearing two women talking about Robert's mother that day. One said, "I hope that Wadlow boy's mother has a good washing machine." The other woman said, "It would take half a clothes line for his sheets." Bentley said she always found it interesting the two women were so con-cerned for Addie Wadlow's washing problems.

On Robert Wadlow's 16th birthday, he was 7 feet 10 1/2 inches tall and weighed 365 pounds. He grew less rapidly in this year than previous years, only gaining 2 1/2 inches and 20 pounds.

Robert almost forgot about his 16th birthday on Feb. 22, 1934. "I don't know whether I'll have a party or if there will be a birthday cake on my birthday," he said before the big day.

Robert had changed his mind about his future career from the previous year. Earlier, he said he wanted to be a lawyer, but now he thought he might do better in the advertising branch of the shoe business.

Robert wanted to go out for basketball at Alton High School, but getting athletic shoes his size was next to impossible. Ray Jackson, athletic director and basketball coach at Alton High, had to constantly explain why Robert wasn't a member of his team. Jackson's normal response was that he was afraid Robert would get hurt.

"We'd take him along to games with us, but we had difficulty finding shoes to fit him," Jackson said.

"I ordered a pair of gym shoes, but it was such a big job that by the time the shoes were finished the basketball season was over," Robert said at the time. "I may use them next fall, if they still fit."

Some thought Robert could have been an excellent basketball player, but he simply didn't have proper coordination for the game with his massive body and large feet.

Gene Crivello first met Robert in 1935 when the pair were members of the intermediate group of boys 14 through 17 years old at the Y.M.C.A. The intermediate program, which included basketball, reading, track and swimming, took place during summer vacation. "Basketball was too cumbersome for him," Crivello said. "He was good at standing at the end of the court and dropping the ball through the net."

Robert ended up having two birthday cakes on his 16th birthday. One was baked by his mother and the other by a friend. He received cards from all over the world.

On Oct. 3, 1934, Robert topped 8 feet tall and weighed 360 pounds. Robert turned 17 on Feb. 22, 1935, and he stood 8 feet

1 1/2 inches tall and weighed 370 pounds. He slept in a bed that was 8 feet long, causing him to bend his knees, and under blankets sewn together. Robert wore a size 36 shoe at 17, increasing from 35 the previous year.

Robert liked the popular cartoon character Popeye but didn't follow his advice of chomping spinach, eating it only sparingly. Reading western thrillers used to be one of his favorite pastimes, but he said he wasn't much interested in those at this point in his life. At the Y.M.C.A. pool at Third and Market streets in Alton where he occasionally swam, Robert walked in the deep end of the pool and kept his head above water without straining. The pool was 7 1/2 feet deep. He employed the "dog paddling" technique of swimming to get around the pool. The boys also played pool and Ping Pong at the Y.M.C.A. A pool cue looked like a pencil in his hand, Crivello said.

When Robert was swimming, he and the other boys had to be very careful, Crivello said.

"He would get in at the shallow end, walk around, and before you knew it, he was in 7 feet of water," Crivello added. "If he lost his balance and fell in the deep end, there was no way he would recover and there was no way we could have gotten him back up. We had to be very, very careful when he was swimming and careful with the other boys making waves while he was in the water. The other kids were very cognizant of the fact he was uneasy on his feet."

Stan Robens saw Robert used at the Y.M.C.A. Pool as a "diving board." Crivello can still picture Robert Wadlow's large, swollen feet. "They were so grotesque," he said. "He wore a size 28 or 29 shoe size at the time. He didn't have any coordination whatsoever. He enjoyed playing with all the guys, though."

Crivello's friendship with Robert was deep. Today, hardly a day passes that he doesn't think about his childhood pal.

Chapter 5

Land Of Giants

Robert Wadlow suffered an infected toe in late March 1935 and became seriously ill. About a week later, he was not showing much progress after being treated with an antibiotic. He was admitted to Barnes Hospital in St. Louis. With a height of 8 feet 1 1/2 inches and weighing 375 pounds, it took eight men to carry him on a stretcher and place him in the ambulance.

On April 1, 1935, it was reported in the Alton Telegraph: "Robert Wadlow Is Improving at Barnes Hospital." Another Telegraph headline on April 13, 1935, read: "Robert Wadlow Still Weak from Long Illness." "Arthritis, from which Robert Wadlow has suffered the last 10 days at Barnes Hospital, where he is a patient, is still causing him a great deal of pain," Mrs. Harold F. Wadlow, his mother, said today. "The ailment for a while affected Robert's hip but has left that quarter and moved to his knee and to the foot, where an infection has set in. Failure to take much nourishment during the last three weeks had greatly weakened the youth, his mother, said today."

On April 17, 1935, the Telegraph finally reported some good news about Robert, saying that he might be home for the Easter holiday. Robert was weak from the infection, having lost 60 pounds.

On May 6, 1935, Robert returned to his home on Brown Street. "He has a good appetite again and may eat anything he desires," Addie Wadlow told the Telegraph. "Of course, he is not yet able to walk again, but Robert is happy to be home, and we are equally happy over his return." The nine-week illness caused Robert to miss graduating with his class at the Alton High commencement in June. Robert then planned to enroll at Alton High in the fall to complete his high school degree work.

After a successful recovery, Wadlow did return to high school in September. During that summer Robert spent some time in Sportsman's Park, home of the St. Louis baseball Cardinals in that day.

Lonnie C. McGiffen once observed Robert and a girl attending one of the carnivals that came to Sportsman's Park in St. Louis. "The carnival owners would allow them to ride free, because with Robert Wadlow on the rides, he attracted a big crowd. I collected tickets for the rides. Robert and his friend especially liked the 'Caterpillar.' It was a ride that had a green top that came down and covered you."

Another time, McGiffen was at Sportsman's Park and a bearded religious group, "The House of David," arrived to play a game against the local squad, the Alton Blues. Many of the Alton Blues team members worked at Owens-Illinois, a glass manufacturing company and other local factories. "The House of David" group was a barnstorming team that toured the country. Most of the barnstorming teams had gimmicks. Each player on "The House of David" club sported beards. Beards for men were relatively uncommon in the 1930s, so it made the team unique.

One night the House of David team came to St. Louis on a bus and parked inside Sportsman's Park. When they all got off the bus, the enormous Robert Wadlow, with a false beard, got off the bus, too. Alton's giant worked as the bat boy for the

House of David club. Since they were afraid Robert would get hurt, they had McGiffen pick up the bats and balls and throw them to him.

Every time Wadlow came out of the dugout to pick up what McGiffen threw over to him, the crowd erupted in a huge cheer. Robert was starting to understand his fame was much broader than just his hometown. He was becoming a nationally recognized figure.

June Pitts Bassford was a classmate of Robert's at Alton High School. She was in Robert's history class taught by Verla Lampert.

"The students accepted him as one of them, not as a curiosity," Bassford said. "Bob was an excellent student and always participated in class discussions. He was always surrounded by his many friends, and he was a very outgoing, personable and fun-loving individual. Whenever he was teased, he teased right back. I don't know how many times his classmates would say, 'Bob, how's the weather up there?' He was always patient and smiling, never seeming to mind."

Occasionally, Robert fell in the Alton High halls and was unable to get up by himself. When that occurred, a group of male teachers and well-built students would line up on each side of him and lift Robert to his feet.

Bassford once double dated with Robert. The occasion was a Christmas party at the Lancaster School of Expression, which Robert and Bassford's dates attended as students.

"I especially remember the trouble Bob had fitting himself into the back of my friend's car, having to bend over double with his chin on his knees," Bassford said. "Since it was a very cold night, all the guests wore hats. One of the boys could not find his hat when it was time to leave the party. We all joined in the hunt, but could not find it anywhere. Suddenly we smelled something scorching and traced it to the high chandelier in the living room.

Robert laughing, easily retrieved the hat where he himself

had hidden it."

Don Lawrence was two years younger than Robert and attended school with him. "We all knew he was big, but we just treated him like any other boy. As Robert grew older, he developed a slur in his speech, and before his death, it became difficult to understand him."

George Louis Mueller was in the Boy Scouts at the same time as Robert. Mueller also went to high school with Robert.

"I remember in high school, in every one of his classes he had to have a special chair because he was so heavy," Mueller said. "They had to enlarge the doors so he could get in and out."

Robert Landiss remembers Robert Wadlow having his individual way during high school.

"Robert didn't have a lot of strength in his feet," Landiss said. "Everybody liked Robert. I remember trading stamps with him outside class before the next class and the bell ringing and him saying he wasn't through yet even though the bell had rung. Robert liked everybody."

Nick Perica had an interesting Alton High cafeteria experience with the world's tallest man. When Perica had a hard time getting in the cafeteria because of a daily lunch time crowd, Perica's sister, Mary, had an idea for him.

"Mary said Robert opened up the hall when he walked through it," Perica said. "She told me to get behind Bob and he would clear the hall for me. I waited to get behind him at lunch and sure enough, he opened everything up and I got in to eat. Bob didn't know what he had done for me. Bob reminded me of a tank."

Perica recalls it being hard for Robert to get to and from class to class. "It took him five minutes to get from his different classes," Perica said. "He sure had some feet on him. I also remember Robert giving his leftover pencils to my friends. Once they got to a certain size, he couldn't use them."

Earl Thomas Griesbaum was the shortest person in the 1936 Alton High School class at 4-foot-10. He offered quite a contrast to the 8-foot-plus Robert Wadlow. Griesbaum remembered sitting by Robert in English class and the two were reciting work from William Tell.

"Robert had a translated version of William Tell in his hand, and his hand was so big we both could see it," Griesbaum said. "The teacher was sitting right there about 10 feet away but didn't see it. I had no intention of cheating. He was like most of our other classmates; he was just big. We were both freaks; I was only 4-foot-10 and he was 8-foot-plus."

Griesbaum possibly bonded more with Robert than nearly anyone else because of their size discrepancies, although they were nearly 5 feet different in height.

"I was the smallest in class and also a left-handed person in a right-handed world," Griesbaum said. "We were both living in a world built for average people. Everyone respected him just as he had respect for everyone else. He knew he was abnormal, but he could have been one of the best psychologists in the world. When in public, he didn't mind because he was observing human behavior more than the public was observing him."

Everett Watson and Robert Wadlow took a photography class together. The class was difficult for Robert, although he loved taking pictures. "As big as his hands were, he had trouble operating a camera," Watson said.

Evelyn Cannon was in Robert Wadlow's German class in high school. Robert struggled somewhat with the language because of his guttural tone of voice. His voice had a harsh, grating sound to it, she said. In fact, it sounded as if Robert's voice had to travel several feet through a hollow tube before it came out of his lips.

"Robert's vocal chords were enlarged, so German was hard for him," Cannon said. "But he worked at it and he was able to pass the course without too much difficulty."

A total of 88 pupils received their high school diplomas on the evening of Jan. 24, 1936, including 17-year-old Robert Wadlow. At graduation, he planned to enroll at Shurtleff

College in Alton in pre-law.

As Robert prepared to graduate from high school, he was regarded by his classmates as a gentle, relaxed individual. Robert admitted hitting only one person in anger despite incessant attention. One burly fellow had pulled up Robert's pant leg and pinched his leg, thinking Robert was on stilts.

"I didn't hit him very hard," Robert confessed. "But he stopped bothering me."

Robert's high school graduation gown required 13 3/4 yards of cloth as compared to a normal 6 yards for other graduates. The gown sleeve was 55 inches long, and the gown measured 83 inches from the collar to a point 7 inches from the floor. The skirt of the gown was 8 1/2 feet around. The size of Robert's cap was 8 5/8.

Robert graduated from Alton High School standing 8 feet 4 inches tall. It is now speculated the height of Goliath, in biblical times, might have been about 9 feet 4 inches. Og, the king of Bashan, slept in a bed that might have been 13 1/2 feet by 6 feet. Porus, an Indian king, who fought against Alexander the Great in 327 B.C., is described as 7 feet 6 inches tall. Charlemagne, who could squeeze together three horseshoes at a time, is listed at nearly 8 feet.

At the time of his high school graduation, Robert Wadlow had a recorded height greater than any other giant accepted by the medical profession. One other man, known simply as Turner in medical documentation, stood 8 feet 3 inches tall. It was noted in a medical volume that Turner was crippled and hence somewhat stooped.

Robert had been able to live a normal life during his first 18 years despite his incredible size. The next stop for Alton's boy giant was Shurtleff College in Alton, where he planned to pursue another of his dreams — a law career. There was still no end in sight to his enormous growth.

Chapter 6

College Bound

When Robert Wadlow turned 18 on Feb. 22, 1936, a newspaper story was sent to 1,200 U.S. newspaper editors by The Associated Press. Most of the nation's newspapers published the account the next day about Alton's amazing young man who stood 8 feet 4 inches tall and weighed an astonishing 390 pounds. The article was about a Gentle Giant and his overactive pituitary glands. Medical science attempted to explain the growth of the 8-footer in interviews to the media.

Robert celebrated his 18th birthday enrolled as a freshman at Shurtleff College in Alton. He had gained only 2 1/2 inches in height from the previous year and thought, "it's about time I stopped growing."

He smiled easily at age 18 and had a low, husky, voice. At the time, his height bothered him because he had to stoop to avoid brushing his head against electric light fixtures.

Times remained tight throughout the United States and in Alton because of the Great Depression, but people looked for heroes and celebrities. Movie stars, gangsters and boxers were glorified and worshipped, and, right along with them, Robert was becoming one of the nation's biggest celebrities.

People were continually asking Robert how much he ate. He wasn't ready to answer that question for the world. "How much I eat or what I eat is nobody's business but my own," he said. "That's the way I feel about it, and it makes me sore every time anybody talks about it." Robert and his family refused to let the public make him a freak show or circus attraction, despite everyone's curiosity.

"As far as circuses are concerned, I wouldn't join one if it was the last thing on earth," Robert said. "There are too many people who stretch their necks at me now."

Robert, eager to learn, took a one-week sabbatical between high school graduation and beginning life as a college freshman. When Robert graduated from high school he didn't want to enter college immediately and thought he might return to high school for a post-graduate course. The high school, however, already was filled at capacity with undergraduate students, with a number of post-grads. So Robert didn't re-enter. After a week at home, Robert decided he had to find something to do and entered Shurtleff College.

Robert remained physically weak from his illness of the previous year and during inclement weather was forced to take a cab to attend Shurtleff classes. He would have walked from his home in Upper Alton to Shurtleff if he had not been so physically drained.

Robert was never one to give up easily on things people told him he couldn't do or achieve because of his size or shape. The German language, looked upon as one of the most difficult subjects for any student at the time, was his favorite subject at Shurtleff College. "I did my best in the thing they told me I couldn't do," he said.

Robert included a German class in his first semester program at Shurtleff College. He earned a course grade of B during two complete years of German in high school. The Alton giant also took courses in political science, botany, English and history during his first semester at Shurtleff.

Quaint Shurtleff College, was founded in 1827 by a pioneer in Baptist ministry, the Rev. John Mason Peck. The institution was first known as Alton Seminary, then Alton College, and in 1853, Benjamin Shurtleff of Boston gave $10,000 to ensure its success, and the college was named after the benefactor. The campus occupied 12 wooded acres of land in Upper Alton in the 1930s when Robert Wadlow attended his freshman year.

Mary Alice Keirle attended Shurtleff College. She was not in school at the same time as Robert but saw him in Upper Alton during his college initiation.

"Robert was five and a half years older than me," said Keirle. "One of the traditions for initiation as a Shurtleff freshman was to wear green beanies. I remember seeing Robert at Block's Ice Cream shop in Upper Alton with his green beanie on. It looked like a little pea on top of a mountain. He went right along with whatever the other kids did, though."

Leonard Bethards wasn't in any of Robert's classes at Shurtleff but often saw him on campus. Bethards said Robert had a hard time with his size at the college and it was difficult for him to travel from class to class. "I remember him slowly taking one step at a time and moving his feet sideways up and down on the steps at Shurtleff College," Bethards said. "I knew Robert's sister Helen really well. We lived at 917 Milton Road, close to Robert's house, so we saw him in the neighborhood all the time."

Robert neared the world's record for height as he started classes at Shurtleff, towering 8 feet 5 inches. Doctors at the time thought he might exceed 8 feet 6 inches if his hyperactive pituitary gland continued to malfunction.

Claims have always been made of circus giants as great as 9 feet tall. These comparisons to Robert usually fell short upon further investigation. The closest documented rival to Robert was the Irish giant Charles Byrne (O'Brien) who an authority asserts was more than 8 feet 4 inches tall when he died in 1783 at the age of 23. Byrne's skeleton was preserved in the Royal College of Surgeons in London.

Among the 18th Century giants were Henry Blackmer, the English giant, and Daniel Cajanus, the Swedish giant. Cajanus was 7 feet 8 inches tall, while Blackmer was 7 feet 4 inches. Chang-wood-goo, the Chinese giant, was reported to have reached 8 feet. Anna Swan, the Nova Scotia giantess, supposedly reached 7 feet 5 1/2 inches in the 1870s.

Alton was divided roughly into five sections in the late 1930s: North Alton, Upper Alton, Middle Town, Downtown and the East End, all separate settlements when Alton was founded. In the 1930s and 1940s, everyone went Downtown and shopped. At that time in Downtown Alton, the busiest places were Sears, Woolworth's Dime Store, Kresge's Variety Store and Snyders Department Store. A Vogue clothing store for women, the Coney Island Restaurant, soda fountains, a grocery store, the Grand Theater and ice cream shops were also downtown. In Upper Alton in the 1930s and 1940s, Harold Jr. recalls another dime store, a pharmacy, Kerr Drugs, Uptown Theater, an ice cream store and Harold Sr.'s Wadlow Shoe Store. Harold Wadlow Sr. ran the shoe store for several years before he was elected mayor. When he became mayor, he didn't have time for the store.

Robert and his family would go to Uptown Alton Theater nearly every Friday or Saturday night and for a quarter, see two movies. Many residents in the late 1930s would spend Friday or Saturday evenings along the Alton Riverfront, watching boats go through the Lock and Dam from a viewing platform. The Mississippi River was always a daily part of Alton people's lives.

Alton was a small town in the 1930s with a population in the mid-30,000s much like it is today. At the time, industry was starting to expand outward. Roxana's Shell Oil and Wood River's Standard Oil had established a presence in the area in the early 1900s, along with East Alton's Western Cartridge Co., a maker of ammunition. Most of the people in the communities worked at the refineries. At one time Owens-Illinois operated the largest glass manufacturing plant in the world in Alton.

Henry B. Lenhardt, now deceased, had a memorable summer experience involving a corn cob pipe with Robert in June 1936 while attending The Order of DeMolay conference in Kansas City, Mo.

"As the Alton chapter was the largest of all at the time, we took a bus load over," Lenhardt wrote. "Robert was among the group, and we met in front of Franklin Temple with a Greyhound bus. There is a picture showing us all lined up. We stopped for lunch in Boonville, Mo. When everyone paid their lunch checks, the owner gave Robert a genuine 'Missouri Meerschaum' pipe, a corn cob with a long curved stem."

Robert fell in love with the corn cob pipe and carried it with him around Kansas City. "As if his size wasn't enough, the pipe really made him stand out," Lenhardt said. Among those attending the DeMolay conference was legendary entertainer/movie producer Walt Disney, who had been one of the earliest of the DeMolays. During the conference, Disney had to take a back seat to Alton's giant.

As Robert Wadlow started college, offers poured in to travel abroad and throughout the country. Two offers were made for theatrical appearances in Europe. One came from London. Others came from Canada and Switzerland. The Berne, Switzerland, offer included a year's tour of Europe.

On July 13, 1936, the Alton Telegraph published an article that said, "Wadlow Tops 'Em All — Now 8 Feet 5. Robert Wadlow, Alton's tall boy, has added more inches to his height according to his mother, Mrs. H.F. Wadlow, of 3204 Brown St. Robert is now 8 feet 5 inches tall and weighs 420 pounds. The Associated Press in checking into its records found that no tallest man living topped the height of 8 feet 5 inches, so Robert is now unique among the tallest persons living."

The Telegraph also carried a newspaper account Aug. 17,

1936, from the London Daily Sketch that said: "Wadlow Weighs 30 Stones Says London Paper."

"At Alton, Illinois, U.S.A., lives Robert Pershing Wadlow, aged 18. He is 8 feet five inches in height — and is still growing! He weighs 30 stones, five pounds and when the height figures are officially verified they will probably prove him to be the tallest human being in medical history. His father, an engineer, weighs a mere 10 stones and five pounds."

In September 1936, Harold Sr. negotiated a contract for Robert to make a nationwide tour of theaters, schools and concert halls. The contract provided that Robert would not appear in carnivals, circuses or in so-called dime museums.

On Dec. 31, 1936, The Telegraph published a story with the headline: "8-Footers Plus Meet and Fuss in Alton."

"If Alton's big boy, Robert Wadlow, had not been a peace loving youth and had lost his temper, there might have been the strange spectacle of a battle of two young eight foot plus giants on East Broadway Wednesday evening when Gilbert "Tiny" Reichert, a close runner up to Bob for height, attempted to pick a quarrel with the Alton boy."

The story in the Telegraph continued: "Reichert, who is 8 feet 1 and much older than Wadlow, is traveling with a basketball team of the House of David, which was here to play the Apex basketball team at Milton School Wednesday. Bob Wadlow, home to spend Christmas with his parents and to let Santa Claus lavish evidences of fond esteem on him, was leaning his 8 foot 5 inches length against a telephone post on East Broadway waiting for a bus to come along to carry him where he wanted to go. While he was standing against the post, up to him came 8-foot-1-inch high Gilbert Reichert. Looking up in the face of Bob Wadlow, Reichert demanded to know what Bob meant by telling around stories that Reichert was not as tall as he claimed to be."

"What makes you tell that I am only 7-feet high," Reichert snapped, "when I am an eight footer."

Robert Wadlow assured Reichert he had never said anything of the kind.

"I didn't even know you were in town," Robert told the other giant. "I have not told any stories about you, and I don't know how tall you are."

Robert, in his typical gentle manner, didn't let the Reichert incident spoil a happy holiday season at the Wadlow home.

When Christmas came that holiday season, Robert received many gifts from near and far. One of the gifts was a fine radio set. Moving about on the Shurtleff College campus (now Southern Illinois University-Edwardsville, Alton School of Dental Medicine) was a chore for Robert. Robert had to go from one building to the next for classes, and it was hard for him to get up and down the stairs. He definitely had the intelligence to fare well in his college classes.

The problem of getting around on campus likely led to Robert's departure from Shurtleff and abandoning his dream of becoming a lawyer. The physical demands were so difficult that he started to think that for the betterment of himself and particularly his family, at least financially, he should go on the road and be paid for others curiosity of him. Many of his college friends thought school was a waste of time for Robert when he could be making large sums of money traveling the country.

The financial pressures of the Great Depression might have influenced Robert's decision to go on the road with his father.

Robert concluded the spring 1936 at Shurtleff, and his report card was not up to his normal standards. If Robert was going to travel the country, he knew he didn't want to do it alone. He needed some sort of manager, and his father fit that bill. Harold would have to leave his 14-year job with Shell Oil Petroleum to travel with his son, but he decided to do it.

When college opened in the fall, Robert stayed home during the first week pondering his next move. Finally, he and his father made the decision it was time to tour the country. One semester of college was all Robert would complete.

Gene Crivello first met Robert in the early 1930s at the YMCA in Alton but later became reacquainted with him in 1936.

"I actually met Robert again at Young's Dry Goods Store where he was doing community service work for tuberculosis," Crivello said. "Robert was sitting in a chair, signing autographs. I was selling shoes next to him. We talked for a long time that day."

Crivello was able to observe Robert eating several times at the YMCA and then later after they became friends again. "Hot dogs and hamburgers were his favorite foods," Crivello said.

Sunshine Rogier took expression lessons with Robert from Mrs. M.S. Lancaster, head of the Lancaster School of Expression. The expression lessons were primarily to prepare students to speak appropriately in public. "I was a teacher at that time," Rogier said. "We had lessons together. Mrs. Lancaster was a nice teacher. There is a picture taken when I was with Robert in class, and that picture means a lot to me."

Harold Shipley had lived next to Robert Wadlow when the family lived on Brown Street in the late 1920s and early 1930s. Shipley also attended Milton School in Alton with Robert. The two didn't see each other again until 1937 or 1938, in Hammond, Ind. Shipley's father transferred to Hammond, and Robert was appearing at Goldblatt Brothers, a shoe store there.

"We went to see him at Goldblatt Brothers since we were old neighbors in Alton," Shipley said. "To my surprise he remembered me."

Paul Breyfogle saw Robert at the Uptown Theater in Alton in 1937-1938. Robert came to the movies, generally on Sunday afternoon. His parents delivered him to the theater in their seven-passenger Plymouth auto. "We placed an ordinary steel-folding chair at the head of the far aisle of the theater where he sat with his long legs extended down the aisle," Breyfogle said. "People quickly learned to maneuver around them. There he enjoyed the show."

About four times a year Robert and his father attended movies at Temple Theater in Alton. When Robert and his family decided to come, the Temple Theater owner Albert Critchlow would issue them free passes and reserve a certain section of seating for Robert. Robert required five seats in the front row of the circle just behind the center orchestra section.

The Temple Theater was unusual with its orchestra group for theater visitors. Most theaters only had movies. He would sit in the center seat of the first three seats on the aisle. His left arm would occupy the seat to the left of him and his right arm the next seat to his right. He would place his legs over the two seats directly in front of him. Those who saw him at the movie theater said this seemed very comfortable for him.

Robert enjoyed going to the movie theaters in the Alton area, but it was always difficult, Harold Jr. said. "Chairs weren't big enough and aisles weren't big enough," he added. "It was hard for him to go to the movies."

Eileen Cunningham saw Robert Wadlow for the first time at a Civilian Conservation Corps Camp in Eldred, Ill., in the mid-1930s. She was visiting the camp while Robert made a public appearance. The CCC camps were created under President Franklin D. Roosevelt's administration during the Great Depression to provide jobs and ultimately food for poor people.

Robert shared the CCC camp members' financial pain during the Great Depression. He thought the appearance might help lift some of the downtrodden people's spirits. Cunningham also saw Wadlow some time between 1936 and 1938 at the Greene County Fair in Carrollton. Carrollton was a small farming community 30 miles north of Alton. "I couldn't believe it was Robert Wadlow at the Greene County Fair," Cunningham said. "He sold his lemonade at the fair and created quite a spectacle."

Later, Cunningham attended Cornell University on the East Coast. Even there she heard of Wadlow in medical lectures and then realized he had gained a permanent place in world medical history.

Robert had grown to 8 feet 7 inches tall by the time his 19th birthday arrived on Feb. 22, 1937. Six months before, Robert stood 8 feet 5 1/2 inches in his shoes, indicating he had grown 2 1/2 inches during that six-month stretch. He had hopes of a dog for his 19th birthday but was traveling a lot away from home at the time. "I thought at first I'd like a wire-haired terrier," he said at the time. "There's one next door, and he's awfully cute; but wire-haireds are so full of pep they're a lot of trouble, so I guess I'd rather have a bigger dog that's calmer; a cocker spaniel is my favorite."

On his 19th birthday, Robert had taken Harold Jr. to see a performing dog earlier in the day prior to The Telegraph's arrival at the Wadlow home for the annual birthday photo. When The Telegraph reporter and photographer arrived that afternoon, 4-year-old Harold Jr. was taking a nap.

"I like to take him places with me," Robert said of Harold Jr.

On the night of his 19th birthday, a surprise party was held for Robert Wadlow. Family and friends gathered at his Brown Street home in Alton. Robert, entering the front door about 8:30 that evening, was greeted with "Happy Birthday To You." Apparently he had been unaware of the planning and mysterious phone calls during the past several days, so the party came as a complete surprise to him.

After the presents were opened, disclosing boxes of candy, handkerchiefs, a camera, three cakes, and flowers, the boys and girls spent the evening telling stories and talking. Robert provided the highlight of the evening telling of his recent trip to Chicago. He also showed his friends a fingerprint book, with his fingerprints on the last page. At age 19, he showed no signs of slowing down in his growth pattern.

Chapter 7

A Devoted Christian

When Robert returned home from his national travels, he spent Sundays at Main Street Methodist Church, where he was a member. The church was a place where Robert always felt at home even if he did stand out like a skyscraper inside the church. Robert began attending the church in the 1930s under the ministry of the Rev. N.C. Henderson.

When Robert walked into Main Street Methodist, it was no different than any other place. Every head turned to watch him walk.

Sunshine Rogier, a lifelong Main Street Methodist Church member, watched Robert in the church setting on Sundays and remembers seeing him having to bend down to get under the balcony.

"When Robert got out of a car, he was so tall, I didn't think he would ever stand up straight," Rogier said. "They had to make a seat on the back row of church for him. Robert's feet went over the back seat of the back row."

James Schmitt and his family sometimes drove Robert home from church on Sunday.

"We took him home in my father, Clarence's car," Schmitt said. "One thing I remember is shaking his hand and his hand covering my whole hand. His hands and feet were so big."

In those days, Main Street Methodist did not have a pipe organ. The Rev. B.H. Batson and Dr. J.E. Walton launched a pipe organ fund drive with Robert at the helm. The plan was to have the organ ready for use and dedicate it on Robert's 22nd birthday.

Robert planned to assist in the fund raising by giving his autographed photograph to every person who contributed. Everywhere Robert went he attempted to raise money to assist his church. Robert sent an autographed photograph to each fund contributor. The organ the church agreed on was a two-manual instrument, with full electric action and cost about $2,000. Once the money was raised, the pipe organ order was placed with Wicks, a famous Highland, Ill., factory.

Harold Jr. described Robert as a good, Christian man. "One of the things Robert was most proud of in his life was chairing the fund drive to buy the pipe organ. He wanted to help the church, and he thought this was a special way he could help."

Robert Landiss attended Sunday school at Main Street Methodist Church with Robert and his sister, Helen. Landiss recalls Robert as being the gentle person he was known for in Sunday school class. "Robert took everything in stride," he said. "He was a happy person all the time."

Vivian Shearburn used to walk with Robert to Sunday school at Main Street Methodist Church. She said Robert was just a regular guy, an ordinary Altonian to most who knew him. Shearburn remembers wanting to connect with Robert while walking to church. Because of his extreme height, the only way she knew how was to reach up and grasp his mammoth hand.

"I also remember him walking up the steps sideways at Main Street Methodist and going in the back door," Shearburn said.

"Robert was a very good Christian. We would laugh and talk each Sunday as we walked to Sunday school. Robert always did the activities that the other people in the group were doing."

Ellen Fenstermann observed Robert Wadlow participating in youth groups at Main Street Methodist Church with one of his sisters. People were always talking about how much Robert ate, and one time she heard him talk about his appetite.

"I remember one time eating, and Robert ordered a hamburger and told his younger brother Eugene jokingly, 'I'll take that one, too, Gene.'"

Another time, Robert joined Fenstermann and her family in a trip to Main Street Methodist. "Robert loved the church," Fenstermann said. "He loved being with young people. Robert was a very good, Christian boy. Everyone noticed him and said hello to him. He was very well thought of in the congregation."

Alice Fisher was a young girl when Robert Wadlow used to labor his giant body into the confines of Main Street Methodist Church. Once, the church was crowded and the only seat available was on Robert's lap. It became something she shared in the future with nearly everyone.

"I was probably 4 or 5 years old when I sat on his lap in church," Fisher said. "I felt like I was sitting high on a stool when I sat on his lap."

Jean Perry lived across the street from the Wadlows on Sanford Avenue in Alton, at 2429 Sanford, while Robert lived at 2416 Sanford.

She remembers seeing Robert with Harold, Jr., holding his hand and walking along Sanford Avenue," Perry said. "That picture will be with me forever."

Bea Teter was visiting her sister one weekend when she went to Main Street Methodist Church and saw Robert Wadlow. Robert had a hot dog in his hand. Robert's hand was so large the hot dog wasn't even visible.

Virginia Weigel was outside several times and witnessed Robert having a hard time getting in and out of the Main Street Methodist Church doorway. There were 15-20 steps for Robert to climb in front of the church.

"I always wondered how many other normal people could cope with all that he had to do," Weigel said. "I remember him coming out of the old church and putting his foot sideways on the steps. His foot was too big to balance."

Jean Garrison was also a Methodist Church member, but she attended a church in Bunker Hill when Robert attended Main Street Methodist in Alton. Garrison's father, Charles Miller, was the Bunker Hill pastor. Charles Miller decided to invite Robert as a special guest to one of their church events.

"At the time, Robert was a great one to have at church happenings," Garrison said. "We tried to get a baseball player or somebody famous to draw a crowd. My dad invited him to come up to a men's supper at Bunker Hill. He came to our house. He was so big and the entryway was so small, he just sat on our steps. I remember how they took half the front seat out of the car for him. It was something to watch him get in a doorway. He was almost bent over double when he went through."

Garrison described Robert Wadlow's voice being "guttural." "It was hard to hear him and understand his words, at times," she said.

Robert's pale skin tone also fascinated Garrison during their encounters. "I remember then thinking he needed some sun," she said. "Robert was so fair skinned and had kind of blondish hair. Robert's fingers were huge. I remember that more than anything, about his fingers."

The original organ Robert helped raise funds for was sold by the church before the Rev. William Fester arrived. However, the chimes were saved and installed on the organ presently in the church. There is a plaque in the church that still reads: "Robert Wadlow Memorial Organ." People from all around the country still gather at the wall dedicated to the history of the church and look at the plaque remembering what Robert did for his church.

Fester said from what he has heard from church members, Robert was a gentle, polite and somewhat shy person. "He was in attendance pretty often at church," Fester said. "I think he did have trouble with the ceiling fans at the church; he had to duck under them."

Main Street Methodist Church named its fellowship hall in honor of Robert. A life-size photograph of Robert by Robert Graul hangs on a hall wall. Sunshine Rogier donated the picture to the church to help preserve Robert's memory.

"Everyone who comes into the hall has to measure themselves up against Robert," Fester said.

Main Street Methodist Church members still gather at many services and chat about the Gentle Giant and what it meant to have him as a part of the congregation. Rev. Fester doesn't think Robert Wadlow will be forgotten for his contributions to the church and the memories of him that have been passed from generation to generation.

Chapter 8

Travels In The Big Apple

Although Robert had said he would never join the circus, he changed his mind in April 1937, signing with Ringling Brothers and Barnum & Bailey Circus. Ringling Brothers had been in contact with Robert for several years to sign. Robert began his travels across country that spring, making contract appearances for Ringling Brothers. The time had come for Robert to earn nationwide billing for his incredible height. Robert's financial needs may have influenced his decision to join the circus even though his father was so adamant against it.

The first stop for Harold Sr. and Robert was scheduled for the Astor House in New York City. The Wadlows' act was supposed to take 10 minutes twice a day and was to be dignified, according to the contract. Robert's performance was scheduled to be the main show with Ringling Brothers.

He stayed for four weeks in New York City and had additional stops in Brooklyn and Boston. The young giant received considerable attention, particularly in the East.

During Robert's eastern travels, he met Admiral Richard E. Byrd and heavyweight champion boxer Jack Dempsey, among other celebrities. Byrd disappointed him, failing to speak of his voyages and undertakings at sea.

Radio stations were frantic to interview Robert during his trip. Robert's visit to the New York Stock Exchange created quite a stir. As he sat in the balcony, suddenly activity on the floor of the Exchange ceased, something that never happened during the frantic daily trading. More than a thousand men gawked his way and trading stopped for a few moments while they observed their Alton guest.

Robert visited the Empire State Building with Mayor Alfred E. Smith as host. New York City photographers caught several shots of Robert in open-top cabs with his large body sticking out.

Robert helped draw a record attendance to Madison Square Garden and Ringling Brothers Circus. He loved getting to see the Statue of Liberty, but his favorite part of the eastern trip was visiting the grounds of the Battle of Concord, a famous Revolutionary War confrontation. "We saw a lot of things there — the place where Americans made their first stand and the North Bridge. I like history so much, that stood out in my mind," he said.

There were three rings in Madison Square Garden during Robert's appearances. When Robert was about to appear, all lights went off and the "spot" was turned on the center ring. Robert walked out into the spotlight and stood for a short time while he was introduced. He didn't have to wear any special costumes.

Initially, the circus people suggested dress suits for him. Harold Sr. told them Robert would wear them if they would furnish some, but they never came up with the suits. Robert stuck to dress shirts, a tie and dress pants for his circus attire, trying to retain his dignity in the appearances.

The New England crowds constantly stared at Robert along the sidewalks. "One man told me I could put a brick on the side-walk, stop and gaze at it for a while and jam traffic in no time at all," Robert said. "I believe it. Dad can talk about those people out there all he wants to. But I noticed one thing. Whenever a crowd like that gathered, he usually was right in the middle of it."

It seemed everywhere Robert went around New York City, a crowd gathered. Once Robert posed for a photograph for a New York City newspaper towering at the same height of a stoplight. Throngs of people surrounded him any time he walked in the already crowded streets.

"We were always running into crowds of people along the sidewalks, looking at something they thought was unusual," Robert said.

During the New York trip, Wadlow was interviewed on WHN Radio Station, New York City. He appeared on the Postal Telegraph Theater Guide's Clifford Adams "Calling All Parties" program. He also visited three radio programs in New York, the Postal Theater Guide on WHN, one in the Empire State Building, and another on Radio City's Bob Ripley's "Believe It Or Not."

The dialogue of the "Calling All Parties" radio interview went like this:

Clifford Adams: "Now, in contemporary time, there is no reason to believe that anyone could top the 8 feet 7 inches of young Robert Wadlow, who has reached the height. And that young man, one of the nicest, modest young fellows you'd ever want to meet, is in the studio tonight as our guest. Bob, the whole wide world is greatly interested in you, and I'm sure they would be interested if we sat down and had a little talk. A friendly little chat between us two. You know, Bob, I'm a great deal more interested in you than the world is because I know you, and I think you are a fine fellow. I've never been out your way in Alton, Illinois, and I'd like you to tell me something of your childhood in Illinois."

Robert Wadlow: "Well, I guess if you let me get started telling about Alton I never could stop because Alton has a great deal of historic interest, and I know most of it."

Adams: "Well, that's splendid, Bob. You just tell me all about it. You know I'm mighty interested in any place I've never visited and doubly so in this instance, as Alton is your hometown."

Wadlow: "I'm warning you, you will have to stop me, because this is something I like to talk about. I suppose I should start off by telling you that Alton is a nice, pretty little town of about 35,000. I know that sounds like a tiny little place to you because New York is so big and has about 200 times that many people. But Alton was the scene of quite a few instances of importance to the history of the United States."

Adams: "Tell me something about them, Bob, I'd like to hear."

Wadlow: "Well, for one thing, Alton was the scene of one of the famous Lincoln-Douglas debates. And also the Lewis and Clark expedition made their headquarters on the outskirts of Alton. Then we have the notorious Elijah Lovejoy. Lovejoy was an abolitionist during the pre-Civil War period."

Adams: "Were there any Indian massacres?"

Wadlow: "No, I don't think there were, but there is an Indian legend about the Piasa Bird."

Adams: "Wow, tell me about that, Bob."

Wadlow: "Well, many years ago, the Indians claimed that there was a big type of bird that nested on the bluffs and whenever Indian braves were going near the bluffs, this big bird would pounce on them and eat them. One day, a courageous young hero volunteered to have himself sacrificed for the Piasa Bird so his tribe could be free of this terrible thing.

"The brave went under the cover of night and placed an ambush on the bluff near where the bird nested. When the morning came, this brave wandered out there alone and unarmed. The bird figured he was a prey and flew down on the bluff and started to feed on him when a sharp arrow killed it. To remember the event, the Indians painted large pictures of the bird on the rocky side of the bluff, and just recently an artist has been there to paint the picture over again."

Adams: "The name of the bird is Piasa?"

Wadlow: "Yes, it's just an Indian name I guess for the bird. I've taken quite a few pictures of it."

Adams: "So you're a photographer, are you? Now that's one of my hobbies. I can see we are going to talk shop about photography for a few minutes. Bob, tell me about what kind of camera you use?"

Wadlow: "I use a German miniature Reflex camera. I have another camera, too, a small camera, but I prefer the Reflex camera because the ground glass gives me a better focus."

Adams: "I agree with you there, Bob. I like that kind of camera myself. Tell me though, have you taken any pictures of this wonderful Ringling Brothers Barnum and Bailey Circus that's packing them in these days at the Garden? You ride in with the circus. It's such a marvelous opportunity to get some grand shots."

Wadlow: "You bet your life on it. I have some very good pictures. It's one of the most thrilling things I've ever seen. When they come flying out over 50 feet in the air on the trapeze I almost get heart failure. I shot several pictures of the trapeze artists."

Adams: "I certainly envy you, Bob, with a chance to take those pictures. You know what interested me, Bob? When I got a chance to see you the other day at the Garden, I saw the Japanese acrobats practicing. I wish I'd had my camera with me then. To tell you the truth, there are so many amazing sights to see at the circus I'd probably used up 50 feet of film and gone broke in one afternoon."

Wadlow: "I feel that way about things, too, even though I'm a part of it."

Adams: "I bet when you were real young you played circus too just like everybody."

Wadlow: "Yes, I did. I think every kid does. We used to put the cabinet over the soap box and make believe it was a tiger. I used to get an old horn and make believe I was a band."

Adams: "Now Bob, tell me a little bit about yourself. About school and other things."

Wadlow: "I'm afraid I used to take advantage of my height while in school. Before I can remember I used to play on the basketball team. Naturally I was the high scorer. But I was 11 years old and stood 6 feet 7 inches. It was an easy matter for me to stand near the basket while others on the team passed the ball to me. I could just reach up a little bit and drop it in. Used to be I was the 'dropper.' I wasn't very accurate for shooting the basket from any other part of the court, but I never missed from close up."

Adams: "I don't see how you could have, Bob. How did you like school, study time?"

Wadlow: "Well, all right, I study all right. I took Latin; that's my language course in high school. But after one term I changed to German. I got along real well in that language. Now I can read a German newspaper very easily."

Adams: "Well that's fine, Bob. Because of your size in school, did they ever have to make special seating arrangements for you?"

Wadlow: "Well they did in grammar school. I had a specially built chair. But not in high school because I had to move around from class to class."

Adams: "How tall were you when you entered high school, Bob?"

Wadlow: "Oh, around 7 feet."

Adams: "When you completed your high school courses how tall were you then, Bob?"

Wadlow: "Eight feet four."

Adams: "You are of great height Bob. I realize all your clothes have to be made to order. How much material does a tailor have to use?"

Wadlow: "Today he uses between nine and a half and 10 and

51

a half yards of cloth."

Adams: "And your shoes, Bob. What size shoes do you wear?"

Wadlow: "I really don't have a size. It's too big for that, but on the base to bottom of the shoe it is around 36."

Adams: "By the way, Bob, you are 8 feet 7 inches in height? What is your present weight?"

Wadlow: "Well I don't know the exact figure, but it is somewhere around 450 pounds."

Adams: "Man, that's pretty big. Now I wonder if you could tell me about your brothers and sisters, Bob. How many do you have in all?"

Wadlow: "I have four in all. Two sisters and two brothers. The youngest of the four is Harold Jr. He is only four and a half years old. He is a real pal, now. He and mom are coming in this week to see Dad and I. He's coming in either Thursday or Friday. That will be nice.

"That little brother of mine is just as bright as he can be. We were in Chicago for six weeks this winter and started talking about the train tracks. My little brother said he didn't care anything about trains, that he already been ridden on one and that he wanted to ride on an airplane next. I have flown a number of times. I enjoyed the trip to New York this time very much. I think it has any other type of traveling beat by a long ways, and TWA (Trans World Airlines) does have some very pretty hostesses."

Adams: "Well, I've never flown, so I have to take your word for it. Tell me, Bob, are you going to stay with the circus or are you going back to school?"

Wadlow: "I'm going back to school probably next fall. Right now I'm a freshman at Shurtleff College. I intend to finish my college course and quite possibly take up law."

Adams: "That's a grand ambition and I wish you every success at it. And now I'm going to say adieu. Our time is almost up. I want to thank you ever so much for appearing in our program. I want to wish you all the luck in the world. Goodbye, Bob Wadlow, and good luck."

As Robert Wadlow walked out of the New York City radio station studio, he realized he was no longer a small town boy from Alton, Ill., but a national celebrity.

Chapter 9

A Doctor's Betrayal;
Westward Travels

When people are 8 feet tall, they spend their lives in the eyes of public curiosity. Robert Wadlow was in the public eye from the time he was a young boy. The Wadlow family allowed Dr. Charles Humberd of Barnes Hospital in St. Louis to visit their home and interview Robert and research his case. To their surprise, the family felt the doctor defamed their son in an American Medical Association report, which was published in The New York Times.

A portion of the report that described Robert as "moody and mean" and "surly, inattentive and resentful" bothered the Wadlow family, especially Harold Sr. The family sued the doctor and the newspaper for libel. The Wadlow family was never interviewed about Dr. Humberd's description and the press flashed the story worldwide. The Wadlow family filed the libel suits as a means to clear Robert's name which they felt had been defamed.

On Jan. 15, 1938, the Wadlow family filed a suit on behalf of Robert Wadlow for $100,000 in damages in the United States

District Court at St. Joseph, Mo. Humberd's article was published Feb. 13, 1937, in the American Medical Journal, the American Medical Society's official publication.

The suit declared that the article was damaging to Robert. The defendant's response raised the point of law that the article was the report of a professional investigation Dr. Humberd had made along scientific lines and to that extent was "privileged."

The doctor's description that Robert was "moody and mean" cut into Robert Wadlow's soul. He was astonished someone would write those things about him. In fact, Robert sat in his room and cried when he read what the doctor had written.

Harold Jr. said the libel suits weren't about receiving financial rewards for the Wadlow family. Basically, the Wadlow family was trying to silence the media when they filed the libel suits.

The Wadlow family said that Dr. Humberd strayed from the truth in some of his details and attributed incorrectly to Robert's characteristics that could not be supported by facts.

More than a month after the first libel suit was filed, Robert celebrated his 20th birthday on Feb. 22, 1938, at his family home in Alton. Robert was 8 feet 8 1/2 inches tall and weighed 460 pounds. He had grown an inch and a half from his 19th to 20th birthday.

Among the guests for Robert's 20th birthday party were former circuit judge Jesse R. Brown, and Alton Telegraph Publisher Paul B. Cousley and his wife, Mary Esther. Guests watched a movie of Robert's U.S. tours and dined on ice cream, cake and apples.

Robert's growth had slowed, but doctors speculated he would continue to grow to 8 feet 9, or 8 feet 10 inches.

The family planned to build a new house to accommodate Robert's needs. The ordinary 9-foot ceilings barely gave him clearance, and he had to stoop going through the doors. The Wadlows' plan was to have high doors. The family planned a special bathtub, high mirrors and different furniture for Robert.

At age 20, shaving hadn't become much of problem for Robert because he still had little facial hair growth. Clothing was a problem, with his shoes stretching to size 36. An advertising contract provided Robert with all his custom-made shoes.

Robert was, of course, a big eater, but didn't have to eat anything special because of his size. For breakfast, he ordinarily ate two eggs, four strips of bacon and a glass of milk.

In July 1938, Robert and his father started a tour westward to the Pacific Coast. The Wadlows visited Cheyenne, Wyo., and attended the last day of the Frontier Days event in Cheyenne at Yosemite National Park. Robert and Harold Sr. saw some of the age-old redwood trees, the tallest and oldest known in the world that dated to as far as Abraham of biblical times.

Next, Robert and his father traveled to Salt Lake City, then by Aug. 8, 1938, were in Reno, Nev. Robert yearned to watch the gambling in Reno and visit some of the much-talked about Nevada clubs.

Their first California stop was in Sacramento, then they left for San Francisco, where the Wadlows stayed for seven days. San Francisco cable cars were an attraction for Robert, and the sight of him in a cable car captivated those in the Golden Gate city.

Robert visited several California valley communities from Sacramento to Bakersfield, including a stint as far south as San Diego. He went out of the United States only once, in early September 1938, before visiting Hollywood. Harold Jr. said Robert asked his father about going a few miles south of San Diego to Tijuana, Mexico, which was just over the U.S. border. Robert's father agreed and the two went to Tijuana shortly thereafter. Robert started walking down Tijuana streets, and a crowd of more than 3,000 Mexicans and tourists surrounded him.

"Robert was invited as a guest to nearly every business in Tijuana that day," Harold Jr. said. "Robert was glad to leave the country."

Next, Robert toured Hollywood and looked forward to his first chance to see if anyone in film circles would be interested in him. Robert and his father arrived in Los Angeles Sept. 11, 1938, and stayed for three weeks at the Biltmore Hotel. "I'm ready and willing," he told the Los Angeles news media when asked about the possibility of a Hollywood offer, obviously hoping to eventually star in pictures.

While in Hollywood, Robert was photographed with movie stars Maureen O'Sullivan and Ann Morriss at M.G.M. Studios. O'Sullivan played Jane in the first "Tarzan" movie, with U.S. Olympic swimming hero Johnny Weismuller as Tarzan. Any other time, O'Sullivan and Morriss made people stop in their tracks and stare, but when Robert was on the movie lot, all eyes were focused on him and his towering height. Robert also visited Warner Brothers Studios.

One of Robert's disappointments on the trip was his visit to "The Jack Benny Show" at National Broadcasting Studios. Robert thought he and his father were going to appear on the show after being introduced to the rest of Benny's cast, but they never made it on the air.

Robert realized that he and Hollywood simply didn't mix. Pat O'Brien and several other cinema celebrities impressed Robert as "nice people," but movie work didn't appeal to him. He said he might have been interested "if I had any dramatic abilities." Robert simply felt after the Hollywood appearance that he didn't have the qualities necessary to make it in Hollywood.

Robert was asked if Hollywood stars worked as hard for their money as people read about and said: "They work even harder than you read about."

Frank Wadlow, one of Robert's cousins, recalls Robert being the toast of Huntington Park, Calif., on his next journey through the West Coast in the fall 1938. There was much advance promotion of the trip as one of Robert's shoes was placed in the window of Gallenkamp Shoes in Huntington Park.

Huntington Park residents filled up the shoe with pennies and were asked to guess how many the nearly size 40 shoe would hold. The winner would receive free shoes during Robert's appearance. Frank Wadlow remembers Robert touring various Gallenkamp stores in California that offered International Shoe Co. products.

When Robert visited Frank Wadlow's home, Frank remembers fearing the giant on his doorstep.

"I was 9 or 10 years old," Frank Wadlow said. "I remember him coming in the house. He scared me to death. He was so tall; our ceilings were only 8 feet. I was completely shocked to see someone that tall. I was asked a lot about him in school because of my name. I took several clippings to school and showed them. I was named for Robert; my name is Frank Robert."

Huntington Park's main street was an elegant place at that time, with a nice residential area nearby. There were many fashionable shops along the street. Today, Huntington Park is a community with a population of nearly 60,000.

"Robert was pretty much a big attraction in California at the time," Frank Wadlow said. "I do remember his father making sure it never became a type of side show. Robert's father and the International Shoe Co. always took care of him. They protected him from being hurt or abused in any way. Each town was always packed with people the day he appeared."

Peggy Timmons, Frank Wadlow's sister, said Robert had to bend to sit on her family couch in Huntington Beach. "I can still remember his legs came up so high when he sat on the couch," she said. "I was just a kid. I remember my dad being thrilled to see him."

From Southern California, Robert and his father embarked on a steamer for Seattle and then went to Oregon. A total of 430,000 illustrated circulars were distributed by Peters Shoe Co. of St. Louis along the westward tour.

Robert enjoyed the Pacific Coast the most of his travels. Oregon, in particular, impressed Robert, and he hoped eventually to make a return trip to Washington. He was dumbfounded by the large Washington redwoods, the largest trees in the world. He told his father that his trip to visit the redwoods was the first time he had ever felt small in his life. Robert and his father left Seattle Oct. 15, 1938, and returned to Alton Oct. 20, 1938. He made a total of 120 appearances.

Robert's 21st birthday party in 1939 was different from most — it was a celebration in which family and guests were joined by the Order of DeMolay in a ceremony to mark his departure from the organization at the Franklin Temple in Alton.

Robert joined the DeMolays when he was 15 or 16 and worked his way up the three degrees before becoming a Mason at age 21. The purpose of the DeMolay organization is providing special activities for youth and serving people. The group has no special charity but strives to help all people in need, whether it is cleaning up a park or taking food baskets to the less fortunate or visiting a nursing home to see a forgotten face. The privilege of serving is the reward for DeMolays.

The DeMolay organization is sponsored and administered by the Masons, but the group was not used as a recruiting station. Many ideals of the two parallel each other, with honesty, brotherly love and high morals.

Harold and Addie Wadlow issued invitations to many family and friends for the DeMolay celebration.

Noll Baking & Ice Cream in Alton offered to bake a big cake and to furnish all the ice cream. The Mothers Auxiliary provided sandwiches and coffee for guests.

Two weeks before the ceremony, Robert was measured at Washington University Medical School. His height in his bare feet was 8 feet 8 1/2 inches and his weight 491 pounds. During the previous six months, Robert had grown three-quarters of an inch and gained 11 pounds. Robert's shoe laces were 96 inches long. Each of Robert's shoes was 18 1/2 inches long, 9 inches in height and weighed 3 1/2 pounds as compared to 1 1/2 pounds of a normal person. It took Missouri shoemakers four times as long to finish a pair of Wadlow's shoes and four times the material of a normal shoe. Robert ordered roughly two pairs of shoes a year at the cost of $100 per pair.

On Feb. 22, 1939, more than 400 attended the 21st birthday party for Robert at the Franklin Masonic Lodge Temple in Upper Alton. First, Robert was honored at the majority ceremony of the Order of DeMolay, a ritualistic program at which a boy, upon becoming 21, formerly withdraws from the order. After that, the crowd went into the banquet hall where the audience and others helped Robert celebrate his birthday.

Two 60-pound, six-tier cakes bore the inscription "Happy Birthday Robert." J.F. Goeken, president of Noll Baking & Ice Cream Co., was photographed with Robert and his father as Robert held a knife to cut one of the cakes. The cakes were the largest that could be baked without special interior supports.

During the Masonic ceremony, Robert was awarded a huge majority certificate, hand engraved by a member of the Masonic fraternity. Robert later heard praise heaped upon him by the other person long considered the tallest man in Madison County, former Judge Jesse Brown, who was 6-feet-6.

Judge Brown drew parallels between Robert and George Washington, whose birthday Robert shared, and Abraham Lincoln, as a product of February and destined to reach great heights. Telegraph Publisher Paul B. Cousley provided quieter praise for the gentle giant. He told the audience that night that Robert had always shown love and obedience to his parents and family.

Brown praised Robert as a man who "has made more friends than anyone I know of" and "one who has lived the most outstanding life of anyone in the world."

"After standing beside you here tonight, I'll never feel so tall again," he said.

Harold Sr. seemed nearly overwhelmed with the round of compliments paid to his son. He answered the comparison to Washington by saying: "Robert has never chopped down a cherry tree, and I haven't been able to get him to chop down any kindling, either."

He also thanked the DeMolay chapter for the massive party and its adviser, J.E. Juttemeyer, and the other groups and individuals who made it possible.

Robert spoke briefly at the ceremony, expressing his modest thanks after presenting a bouquet to his mother, given to him by Juttemeyer, a glorification of the ceremonial flower each newly initiated DeMolay is given to take home to his mother.

Robert Landiss and Bob Rutz were escorts during Robert's DeMolay ceremony.

Landiss, who was 20 at the time, said the DeMolay ceremony was a joyous event in the history of Alton. "Robert was proud that night of being a DeMolay and becoming a member of the Masonic Lodge," he said. "Robert Rutz and I were on each side of him as he went through the different stations that night. I remember everyone taking pictures that evening."

Robert had nearly reached his full height the night of the DeMolay ceremony. Landiss remembers coming up to about Robert's belt buckle. He said those in attendance that night truly loved Robert. "We didn't think of him as a showpiece," Landiss said. "To us he was a normal person. Anybody who knew Robert loved him.

"Robert was a good DeMolay. My favorite memory of Robert is of him being himself. He was an outstanding person. He was very easy to get along with. Robert liked everybody."

Robert may have liked everybody, but the night of his 21st birthday displayed how much the Alton community and people nationwide embraced and held him in high regard.

Chapter 10

Coming To Trial

The $100,000 libel trial for Robert Wadlow against Dr. Charles Humberd of Barnard, Mo., began March 5, 1939, in a St. Joseph, Mo., courtroom. The Wadlows' attorneys filed the case in St. Joseph, because it was a neighboring district court to Barnard.

Robert Wadlow was 8 feet 8 1/2 inches tall when the trial began and weighed 491 pounds. On the first day of the trial, the courtroom was jammed by hundreds hoping for a peek of the world's tallest man. Robert walked into the courtroom with his family for the opening day neatly dressed in a gray suit.

When Robert went from his hotel to the crowded courtroom, he created traffic jams. It seemed everyone in St. Joseph wanted a glimpse of the Alton giant. Crowds blocked the hallways on the third floor outside the council chamber and the first floor lobby when Robert went in and out. St. Joseph police had to plow a path through the crowd for Robert to enter and leave each day.

Autograph seekers were in abundance daily, consisting primarily of school age girls and boys, extending their pieces of paper to the Alton giant. After receiving a signature, the boys and girls left with smiles as big as Robert stood.

A St. Joseph hotel manager had a carpenter take the foot off one bed and the head off another, then splice the two together, head and foot, on the chance Robert would apply for a room, which the Wadlows did.

A number of Alton residents were called as witnesses, including five members of the Alton High School faculty. In the opening round of testimony, Robert denied that he had ever made "pocket money" by charging to let people take photographs of him.

"So many people come around to take pictures of me that we charged them 50 cents for the privilege to discourage them," Robert said in his deposition. Robert testified he could not recall how many times he had posed for newsreels. Dr. Louis H. Behrens, St. Louis internist at Barnes Hospital, who had known Robert since he was 11 years old, denied that Wadlow, as characterized by Dr. Humberd in his article, was the acromegalic type of giant, which causes abnormal enlargement of the head, thorax, hands and feet.

"His hand is very large, but we doctors have gloried in its perfection," Dr. Behrens testified. "He has such a beautiful hand from the artistic standpoint that we have had a cast made for that very reason."

Dr. J.E. Walton, an Alton physician who knew Robert for 18 years, admitted Robert did not have normal ease in walking, but accounted for it by citing the extraordinary length of his leg bones and muscles, which slowed his movements. Mentally, Robert was alert and normal and not "languid and blurred," as characterized by Dr. Humberd, and had always been "very happy and pleasant with strangers and people he met in general" instead of "surly, inattentive and resentful," the Alton doctor testified.

Robert's mother testified in her deposition that she had not approved of many articles published about her son "because they were exaggerated." She said Humberd's allegations that

63

she was resentful of Robert's size were false. She said she was proud of his size.

The following day, March 7, 1939, Robert's family physician and two Alton High teachers testified. Dr. Walton completely differed from Dr. Humberd's article in the American Medical Association Journal that Robert's expression was surly and indifferent. Walton also stated that Robert was not inattentive, apathetic, disinterested, unfriendly and antagonistic as reported by Dr. Humberd.

Two of Robert's teachers who testified were Jane Henry, who managed the school cafeteria in addition to her teaching duties, and Irene Degenhardt, an English instructor. They testified they saw Robert daily and that he responded normally to teaching, ate normally and was a "regular boy." Degenhardt said the only concession granted Robert due to his size was providing a chair larger than those used by other students.

Dr. Walton denied that Robert's attitude was "soured and embittered," as stated in the article attributed to Dr. Humberd. Addie Wadlow refuted Dr. Humberd's comments that her son was "surly, indifferent or otherwise unpleasant in his relations with others." During Addie Wadlow's testimony, her giant son was seated in a chair made especially for his comfort.

She was a private person, so the St. Joseph court appearance was extremely difficult for her. Addie testified that she and Harold along with Robert had objected to Dr. Humberd's examination at the time because it was time for their evening meal and Robert had just arrived home from school with his clothing damp from the rain falling outside. Addie Wadlow said Dr. Humberd did not inform them he intended to write an article about Robert for the American Medical Association's magazine and did not use information he obtained at their home in the article.

When the article appeared in the magazine, Addie Wadlow testified that "Robert cried." She said he also seemed "very depressed for several days."

Cross-examination began on the evening of March 6 and continued during the morning of March 7. The beginning of the cross-examination brought out the fact that the findings of physicians at Barnes Hospital who had examined Robert had been published.

The defense also described Dr. Humberd, the coroner of Nodaway County, Mo., as "the American authority on giantism."

The defense said it planned to establish that the facts of the article as truisms and that the article was privileged since it was written by a doctor of the American Medical Association.

Harold Sr. told the court on March 7 that his son had been a person of public interest since age 9. He said up until the time Robert was 12, he tried to avoid publicity but that since that time he has not objected to being in the public eye. Robert's father said that the articles describing the youth's capacity for food were erroneous and Robert ate only slightly more than an average person.

Dr. David P. Barr, a member of the Barnes Hospital staff, testified it was his opinion that Robert had developed mentally and emotionally as any other boy between the ages 12 and 17.

Counsel for Dr. Humberd called J.R. Erlich, 32, of El Paso, Texas, who testified that the doctor was an authority on the subject of giants. Erlich was 7 feet 6 1/2 inches tall. He also said Humberd had always been kind to him in his writings. Glenn Hyder, 40, of Kansas City, also a 7 footer, said Dr. Humberd had been his friend for six years and always sympathetic to him.

One of the most debated words of the trial was the word in Humberd's Medical Journal article that Robert was an "introvert." Defense counsel argued there was no disgrace attached the word.

Alton Schools Principal C.C. Hanna was called to the stand to discuss Robert's intelligence quotient score of 110, compared to the normal 100. The defense asked him if the intelligence tests had been altered somewhat since Robert's had been given during his junior high years, but Hanna said they still followed the same principles.

On March 9, the jurors met in a downtown St. Joseph theater to watch newsreels presented by the defense. The scenes included Wadlow's 20th birthday party; two scenes in New York City; one in Kansas City; one at the Atlanta Boy Scout camp where he was playing leap frog; and one at Alton that showed him playing basketball. Judge Merrill E. Otis decided to show the films in the theater after deciding it was not feasible for the jury to view them in the courtroom. After the jury had watched the films, court adjourned to the regular courtroom. It took the police a one half hour to unscramble the major traffic jam that occurred when Robert Wadlow walked outside. Everyone wanted to see the giant up close.

After a short deliberation, the jurors returned with a verdict in favor of Dr. Humberd. The Wadlow family accepted the verdict solemnly and filed out of court one by one without emotion, but determined this was not the end of the case. Harold Sr. told the press: "The fight has just begun."

"We will carry that appeal as far as we can," he said, "to the Supreme Court of the United States, if necessary. While we lost the suit at St. Joseph, we feel that Robert was vindicated. The defense testimony was to the effect that no reflection was made of Robert's mental development and that references to his disposition and manner, in the article, were only as of the time of the visit of Dr. Humberd or during the times that Robert was undergoing hospital examination. Most of the time that Robert was in the hospital, he was ill; one time seriously."

On April 4, 1939, Robert, who stood 8 feet 8 1/2, marked his ballot for the first time at a voting booth in Alton Seventh Ward.

He stood more than two feet outside the booth and had to mark his ballot high above the booth against the brick wall. Once again those present in the polling place were captivated, watching the world's tallest man vote. Robert was thrilled to vote for the first time.

On May 9, 1939, the Wadlows decided they would not file for appeal of the Humberd lawsuit. They felt the cost was too much. Judge Otis overruled the motion of Robert Wadlow for a new trial June 19 of that year.

"We are sure that the plaintiff had a trial even more fair than he had a right to ask," the judge said.

Robert appeared on Mary Pickford's Tuesday night broadcast of "We the People" in October 1939 during a trip to New York City. He strongly preferred traveling by plane because of the discomforts he encountered on trains.

Harold Jr. remembered flying on an airplane with his mother to see Robert and his father in New York City. "I was just a kid you know," Harold Jr. said. "It didn't impress me; I was his little brother. All I was impressed by was how he treated me. He was my big brother. He was always kind to me."

On Nov. 5, 1939, Robert became the biggest Mason in the world at the Franklin Lodge. Robert Wadlow and his father received their Master Mason degrees at the Lodge in front of a large crowd. The family tried to keep the ceremony a secret, but word leaked out and representatives from 52 lodges in 11 states attended.

Another Wadlow suit was filed Nov. 6, 1939, for $100,000 against Time, Inc., alleging Robert was libeled by an article in the March 1, 1937, issue of Time magazine. The bill of complaint said the young Wadlow was held up to public scandal, ridicule and disgrace, public hatred, contempt and aversion; his reputation had been impeached, and he had been caused great mental anguish, depression and loss of sleep over the article.

On Dec. 1, 1939, the Time Magazine libel suit was ordered transferred from the Circuit Court of Madison County to the United States Court of the Southern Illinois District. Time Magazine asked for dismissal of the suit in February 1940, and Federal District Judge Charles G. Briggle took it under consideration. On May 6, 1940, Judge Briggle in Springfield, Ill., dismissed the suit.

Harold Sr. did most of the work in the libel suits and pushed to make them become a reality. "Dad was a pretty strong personality," Harold Jr. said. "He knew they wouldn't win when they filed the libel suits. The libel suits were more of a nuisance than anything else."

Harold Jr. said that an apology was what the Wadlow family was actually looking for and when they got it from Time Magazine it went a long way toward helping them cope with the pain created by the articles.

Robert and his father went back on the road for International Shoe, touring the country once things quieted down from the libel suits. Robert was becoming a household name in nearly every corner of the United States.

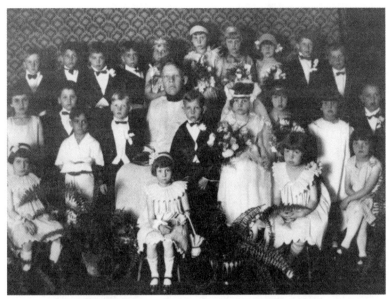

Robert in Tom Thumb Wedding in 1928.

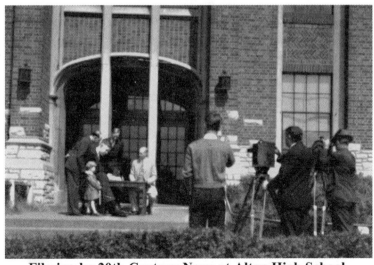

Filming by 20th Century News at Alton High School.
The Telegraph/Robert Graul

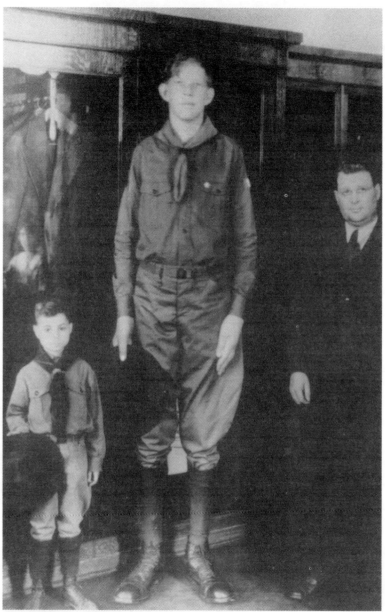

Robert in his Scout uniform with a fellow Scout and Scout commissioner, Hugh Craton.

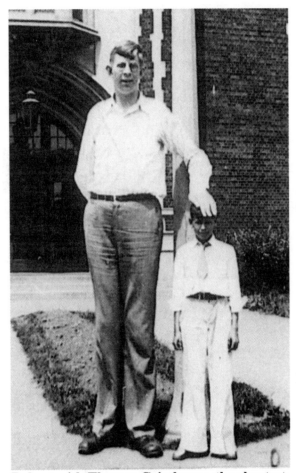

Robert with Thomas Griesbaum, the shortest person at Alton High School in the mid-30s.
Photo courtesy of Thomas Griesbaum

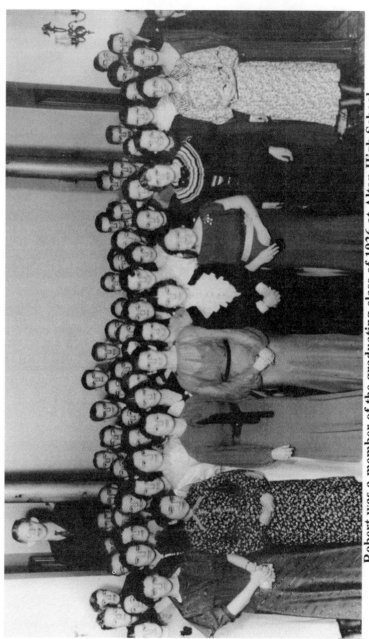

Robert was a member of the graduating class of 1936 at Alton High School.
First published photo of local interest of Robert in The Telegraph by Robert Graul

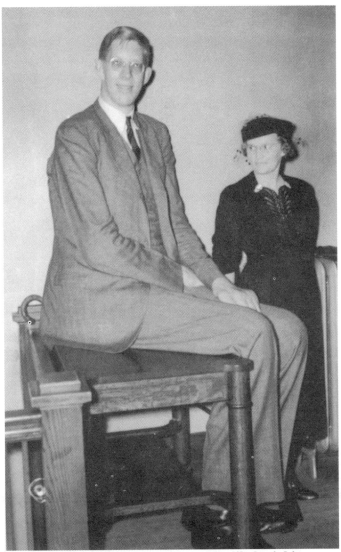

Robert and his mother, Addie, at the libel trial in 1939.

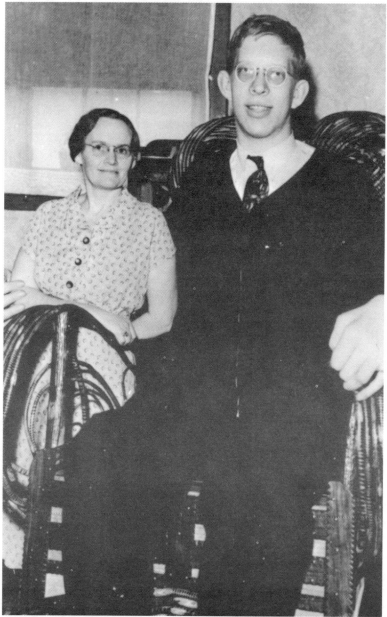

Robert and his mother on his 18th birthday.
The Telegraph/Robert Graul

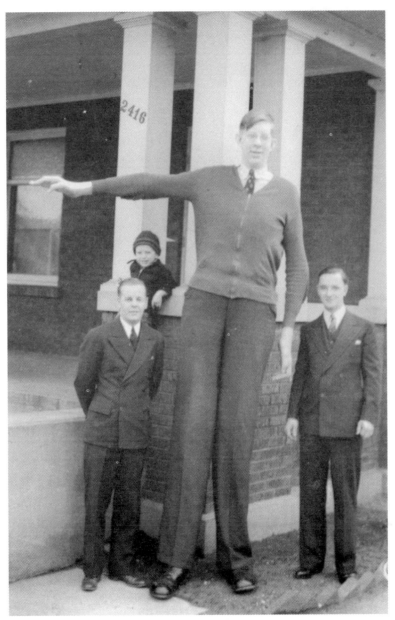

Robert with Harold Jr. on steps and two visitors, Frank Hedger, left and William Graul. *The Telegraph/Robert Graul*

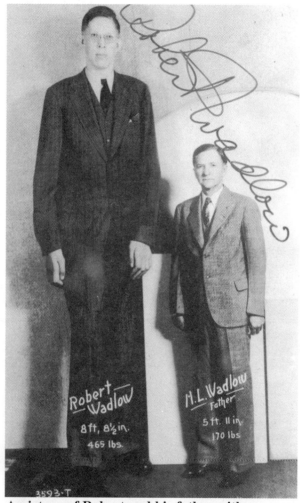

A picture of Robert and his father with Robert's autograph.

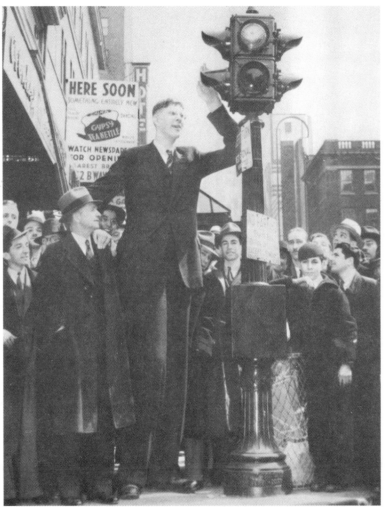

Robert easily reaches the top of a stoplight in New York City while on his U.S. tour.

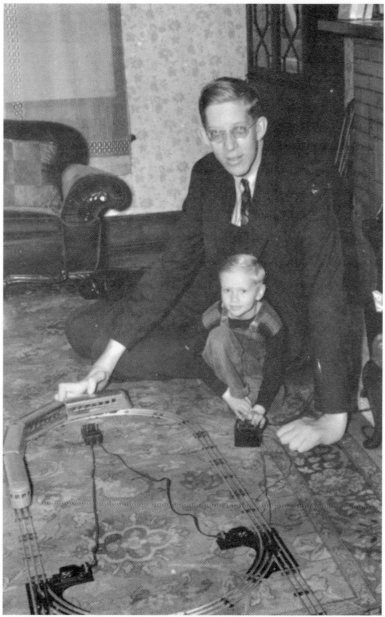

Robert on floor with Harold Jr. in 1939.

The Telegraph/Robert Graul

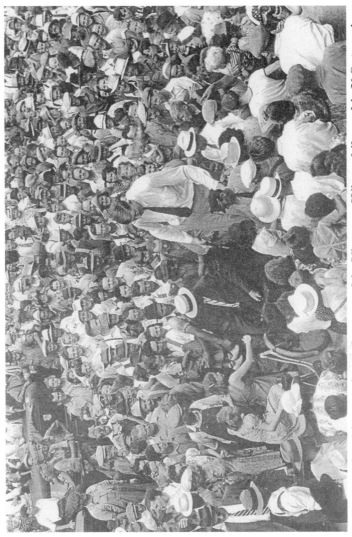

Robert makes his way through a crowd in Viroqua, Wis., while on his U.S. tour in 1939.

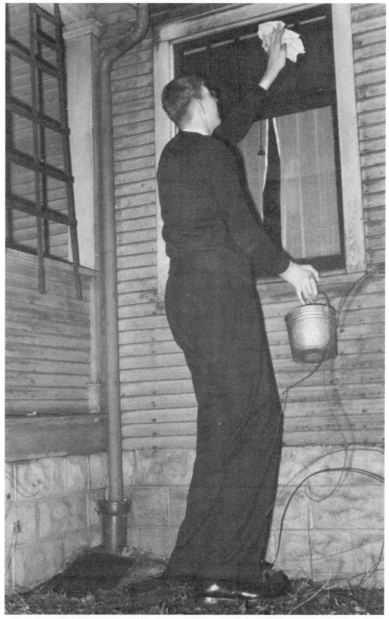

Robert washing a window at his Alton home.

Globe-Democrat photo

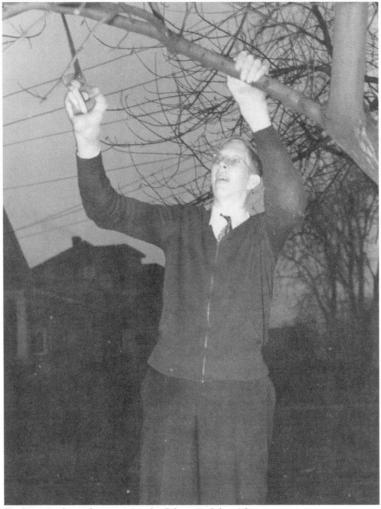

Robert trimming a tree in his yard in Alton.

Globe-Democrat photo

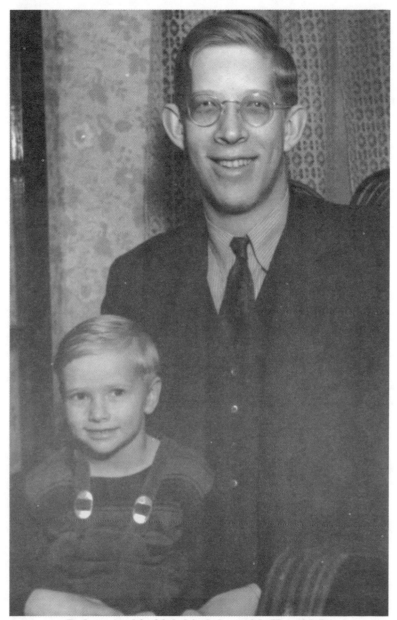

Robert on his 20th birthday with Harold Jr.
The Telegraph/Robert Graul

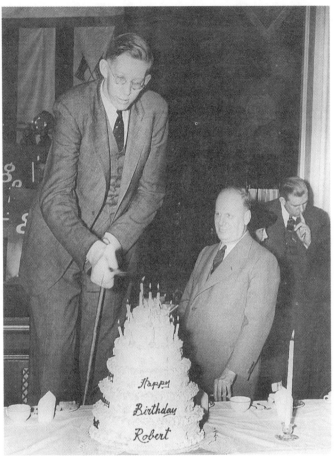

**Robert at his 21st birthday party with Joseph
Goeken of Nolls Bakery.**

The Telegraph/Robert Graul

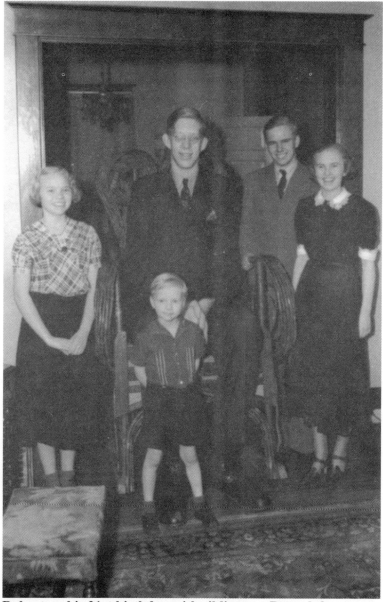

**Robert on his 21st birthday with siblings — Betty, left,
Eugene and Helen — Harold Jr. in front in 1939.**

The Telegraph/Robert Graul

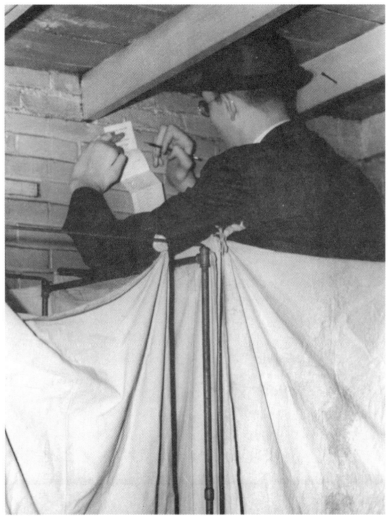

Robert marks ballot in city election, but keeps curtain closed as required by law. *The Telegraph/Robert Graul*

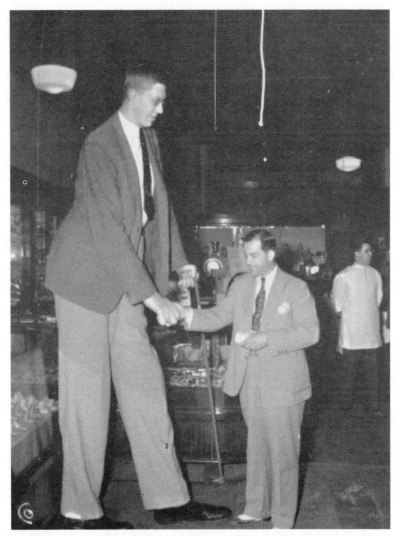

Robert receives his Masonic ring from Robert Goulding at the Goulding's Jewelry Store on West Third Street in April 1940. *The Telegraph/Robert Graul*

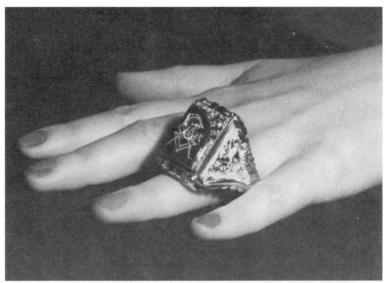

Robert's Masonic ring — a size 25, modeled by Elizabeth Olthoff, clerk at Goulding Jewelry store.

The Telegraph/Robert Graul

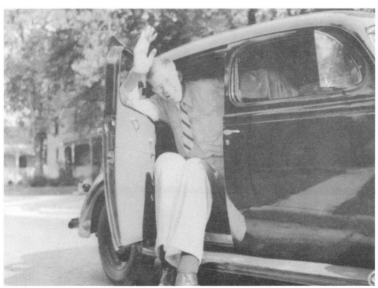

Robert tries out a new Plymouth.

The Telegraph/Robert Graul

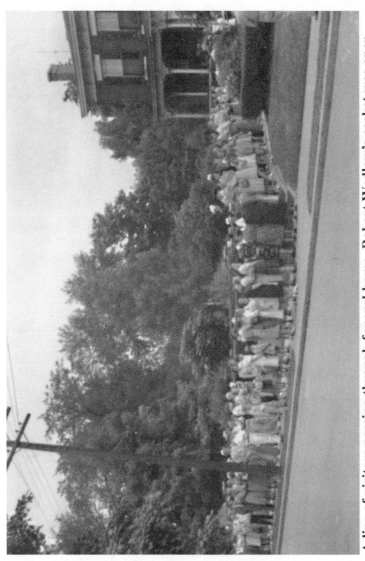

A line of visitors passing through funeral home. Robert Wadlow's casket was open for 36 hours at Streeper Funeral Home (now Elias Smith).

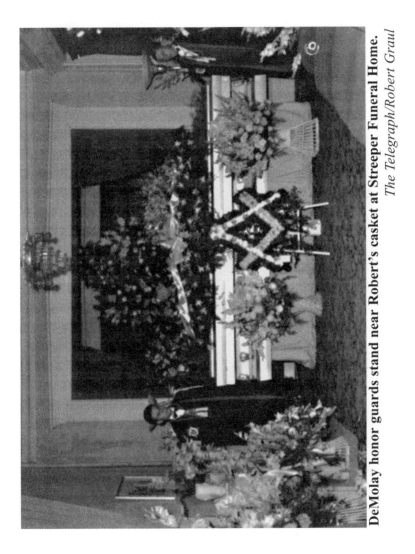

DeMolay honor guards stand near Robert's casket at Streeper Funeral Home.
The Telegraph/Robert Graul

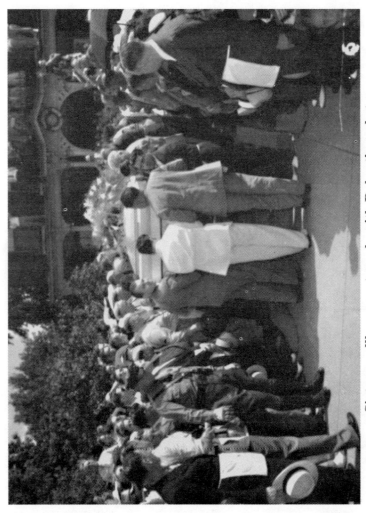

Sixteen pallbearers struggle with Robert's casket.

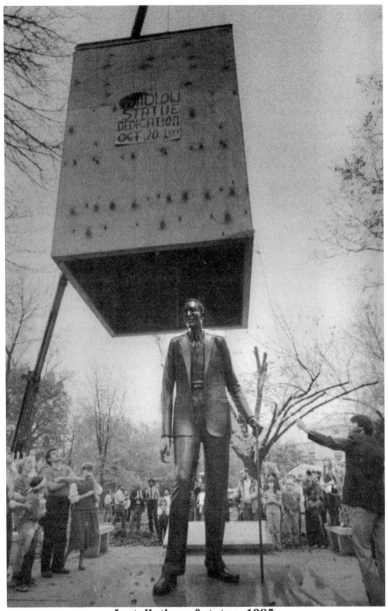

Installation of statue, 1985.

The Telegraph/Robert Graul

Watching Robert Grow

AGE	HEIGHT	WEIGHT
Birth	No Record	8-1/2 lbs.
6 Months	No Record	30 lbs.
1	No Record	45 lbs.
1 1/2	No Record	67 lbs.
5	5'4"	105 lbs.
8	6'	169 lbs.
9	6'2"	180 lbs.
10	6'5"	210 lbs.
11	6'7"	222 lbs.
12	6'11"	241 lbs.
13	7'2"	255 lbs.
14	7'3"	301 lbs.
15	7'8"	355 lbs.
16	7'10"	374 lbs.
17	8"	(sick) 315 lbs.
18	8'4"	391 lbs.
19	8'5"	480 lbs.
20	8'7"	488 lbs.
21	8'8"	492 lbs.
22.4	8'11.1"	439 lbs.

Robert Was Involved

He was a member of the following organizations in Alton, Illinois:

Young Men's Christian Association
Boy Scouts of America
Order of DeMolay
Main Street Methodist Church
Franklin Masonic Lodge

In 1931 he joined the Boy Scouts — if you have ever read a Boy Scout Manual you will readily see what trials would confront a boy of Robert's size.

Robert collected stamps, match books, and rocks, and he also enjoyed photography.

He visited a great many hospitals, schools, orphanages, army camps and charitable institutions.

Robert loved children and he seldom refused a request to visit an orphanage or children's hospital.

Chapter 11

Seeing The U.S.A.

Robert Wadlow started a southern tour of the United States on Feb. 5, 1940. He didn't know it at the time, but most of the rest of his life would be spent on the road away from his hometown.

Robert observed his 22nd birthday on Feb. 22, 1940, at a hotel in Fort Myers, Fla. It was the first birthday he had spent away from his home and family. He and his father planned to visit Mississippi, Alabama, Florida and Georgia on the trip.

Harold Sr. had the hotel in Fort Myers bake Robert a special cake for his birthday. Addie Wadlow was interviewed on Robert's 22nd birthday and said she didn't know if her son had changed in height or weight because he hadn't been measured recently. Robert was 8 feet 8 1/2 inches tall and 491 pounds on his 21st birthday Feb. 22, 1939.

Harold Jr. said Robert enjoyed meeting people and traveling. "He traveled to most of the U.S. states and the small towns," Harold Jr. said. "Robert liked people. I wouldn't be surprised if in the back of his mind he knew he was helping the family financially and at the same time he was traveling with Dad. But the travel was hard on Robert. Dad had to get a seven-passenger car and modify it, removing the front passenger seat so

93

Robert could sit in the back seat and stretch out his long legs. They traveled mainly by car from state to state. Robert was a big kid, but I can't imagine that traveling didn't bother him."

Robert visited more than 800 towns and 41 states. The father and son team traveled more than 300,000 miles on their good-will tour for the shoe company.

Harold Jr. didn't think Robert resented traveling with his father, although some have hinted that it was opportunistic for his father to take him on the road.

"My dad was on salary from the International Shoe Company," Harold Jr. said. "Dad was a good father and a good man. He did enjoy the spotlight that Robert created. Dad had worked around plants until Robert started traveling. Mother and Dad were always very protective of Robert. Most people were just curious about his height, and most people who came to see him were good people. But some did hurt his feelings, making fun of his height. He got to where he could take it."

Harold Jr. remembered Robert as always good-natured about everything. He said his father did most of the speaking when the two traveled across the country.

When Robert was back in Alton, he was accepted as the native son he was in the community. Alton was a small, country town back then, and Robert relished the time he got to spend in the river city. "When Robert got older and was traveling, it was like Robert and my father were on a constant vacation," Harold Jr. said. "They came home for a while from a trip, then they'd get ready for the next trip. Robert sure loved Alton. He sure liked getting back home when he traveled."

Each time Robert returned home he never entered the Wadlow's Sanford Avenue front door without a special toy for his baby brother, Harold. While traveling, Robert was exposed to different colors and creeds. Robert loved people, regardless of their color, even though segregation was strong throughout the country at that time, especially in the South.

"Robert wasn't racist at all; he had problems of his own, so he didn't worry about other people," Harold Jr. said. "Robert lived in a world the rest of us don't understand. He saw and did things we never will do. He met governors, mayors in all the towns he went to across the country. He lived an extraordinary life."

Robert traveled by auto, train and plane. He logged as many as 45,000 miles a year toward the end of his life. One of the things Robert's father had to watch for was Robert peeking into rooms as they walked to their own room in hotels. Robert was so tall that he could see above the glass transoms that were in style at the time.

"Hotel rooms are never private when Bob walks down the halls because he can see through the transoms," Harold Sr. said.

Robert said, "Dad gets mad because I won't lift him up to peek, too!"

A.L. Johnson was Robert's supervisor with International Shoe. He too remembers that about the only problem with Robert in small hotels was that he would occasionally gawk into other people's rooms. Johnson and Robert's father often had to nudge Robert to move ahead when he was glancing into other rooms.

"Robert's life was clean, and he was kind," Johnson said. "He was the kind of boy any mother and dad would be proud to call their own."

Harold Kirsh was a field representative during Robert's International Shoe Co. days. He remembered traveling from town to town with the Wadlows.

Kirsh described Robert as a normal, clean person. Robert was constantly concerned about his appearance and would often have Kirsh inspect him and make sure his tie and shirt were tidy before they made personal appearances. Kirsh also remembers Robert being wonderful with children.

"Robert was never too busy to go to visit with children in schools and orphanages," Kirsh said. "He always took time to be with children."

Robert enjoyed seeing attractive women in their travels and always displayed proper manners and a sense of humor. Girls enjoyed being with him, but Robert never took advantage of anyone with his popularity. Robert had pictures taken with several movie stars during his travels and always was a gentleman around the opposite sex, Harold Jr. said.

"He didn't have much time for girls with all the travel," he added. "He also didn't live long enough to develop a relationship. I don't know if he would have married if he had lived. There weren't many tall women around back then."

Harold Jr. said Robert simply didn't have much peace and quiet. As he traveled the country, he was stared at and stopped nearly everywhere he went, much like a famous movie star or rock star today. Back then, without television, Robert was truly an oddity. Overall, most people were curious about Robert but understanding.

While on the road, Robert liked to dress nice although everything for him had to be specially made. Harold Jr. said Robert was always particular about his ties and shirts and how he looked. When Robert went on the road, he was often put on a flat bed truck at the town stops to sell shoes.

"A local tall boy would come," Harold Jr. said. "They would put him up alongside Robert. People wouldn't believe he was as tall as he was. Dad would put a silver dollar on Robert's head. The local boy would come up and try to touch the silver dollar and could never reach it. No one ever reached the silver dollar as far as I know. Usually, Dad gave the boy the silver dollar for trying."

C.W. Leonard saw Robert Wadlow in his Galax, Va., hometown in 1939 when Robert came to advertise Peter's Weatherbird Shoes for Andrew's Shoe Store on Main Street. It was noon on a weekday when Robert appeared standing on a flat bed truck in front of a large crowd.

"A five-dollar bill was placed on Robert's head, and anyone in the audience who could reach it could have it," Leonard said.

"Back in 1939 five dollars was a lot of money! The only person to try to get the five dollars was Troy Harrison's son, who was six feet six inches tall. When he started up onto the truck, everyone was cheering because they thought surely he could reach the money. But when he reached Robert, he didn't look half as tall as he did walking up there. Needless to say, he did not get the five dollars."

While Robert was in Galax, C.L. Smith Upholstering Co. built Robert a customized chair. The chair with one of Robert's shoes placed on the seat was displayed in the window of Andrew's Shoe Store. Later, the chair was shipped to Robert in Illinois.

The Wadlow chair stood 6 feet 3 inches in height and was 39 inches wide. The width of the seat was 27 inches and the depth was 27 inches. The chair weighed 450 pounds and was made of solid black walnut frame and back posts that were southern red gum. A stock chair is 33 inches in height, 32 inches wide and has a 19-inch seat and is 23 inches deep. Wine colored brocatelle was used for the covering, and 11 yards were required for the job.

"As Robert was leaving, I saw him getting into his car, and it has always puzzled me as to where he put his long legs," Leonard said. "At the time I saw him, Robert was using canes. I'm very glad Robert came to Galax in 1939 and I had the privilege of seeing him in person."

Lane W. Isaak recalls seeing Robert Wadlow in 1937 or 1938 in Kulm, N.D.

"I believe he represented Peters Shoe Co. that day," Isaak said. "He rode on a flatbed in a large chair or bench, pulled by a tractor down Main Street, waving at the crowd. I was about 3 years old at the time. It left an indelible impression on me, and I'll never forget him."

Don Heuer of Batesville, Ark., had the privilege of traveling with Robert's group to Mountain View, and Harrison, Ark., and Branson, Mo. Robert had come to Batesville to visit Heuer's

97

father's shoe store in the mid 1930s. "Dad advertised with circulars delivered town to town by car with boys riding the car's running boards, jumping off to put the circulars on all the porches in a neighborhood," Heuer said. "We covered the entire town. Without radio stations in small towns, advertising was by newspapers, circulars and mouth to ear.

"Robert's visit was advertised in this manner months before his arrival. Thousands of people came to see the Gentle Giant. They walked, rode horses or mules, came by wagons and a few in cars. The street was roped off from corner to corner for people. They treated him with respect, even though a few thought he was not really that tall and that perhaps he was on stilts."

One hot summer day, a dusty country road took the Wadlows to a location in the White River and Sycamore Creek area just west of Mountain View. There they met Heuer's dad's uncle and his family for an afternoon of swimming and to take rides in a johnboat Heuer's father had for the occasion.

"Dad offered boat rides to everyone except Robert," Heuer said. "He was told that if he fell out of the boat there would be no way to get him back in the boat. The rides continued, with fun and visiting taking place, until someone noticed that Robert was missing from the group. They found him on the dusty road trying to thumb a ride back to Batesville. If he could not ride on the boat, he would go back to the hotel. He was told to come back, he would get his ride. I have a picture of Robert on all fours, in that johnboat cruising up the White River."

Heuer's father, brother, nephew and Mr. James from Peters Shoe Co. joined Robert and his father for a trek to Hot Springs, Ark. At the time, Hot Springs was a "mini Las Vegas." The group went to a nightclub where it was required that people attending the show wear a coat or jacket.

"Robert had neither, and it was very hot," Heuer said. "My dad told them we have a young man with us who did not have a coat or jacket and that he was a big boy. He was told, "No problem, we have loaners." Dad said he was a "big boy." They

98

said again, we have big jackets and coats, too. When they saw Robert, they said, "He is a big boy isn't he?" Coatless, Robert was able to see the show."

Robert Wadlow went to the Heuer home for dinner several times. Often he would say to his father, "Ah, Dad, one more piece of pie." When Robert Wadlow stayed overnight in Batesville, the hotel had to put three double beds side by side so Robert could sleep crossways.

"Robert was the world's tallest man on record but also a very easy going guy," Heuer said. "He was a fine fellow and a gentleman."

Delora L. Dunlevy saw Robert Wadlow several times in Springfield, the Illinois state capital, when she was a little girl. One time she saw him at the Orpheum Theater and other times he was simply walking down the Springfield streets. "I remember feeling sorry for him because people stared at him," she said. "His expression was kind of sad looking, and he moved at a slow pace."

Ethan McKay saw Robert Wadlow when he was 9 years old in a visit with the International Shoe Co. to Viroqua, Wis. McKay's father had an International Shoe store in the small Midwestern town.

"Robert was a very friendly and gentle man," McKay said. "One photograph I have shows farmers trying to pluck the five-dollar bill off his head without jumping or standing on their tiptoes. I also remember the local drugstore providing a milkshake to him when he visited and the 'shake' was still in the metal mixing container from the soda fountain. His hand completely concealed the container when he drank from it."

One of Robert Wadlow's stops took him to Decatur, Ill., on Oct. 21, 1939, to eat supper with his family. Wadlow was on his way home from a personal appearance in Morris, Ill., a small community southwest of Chicago.

Wadlow, who was 21 at the time, created quite a stir both inside and outside the restaurant. Onlookers pressed their noses against the restaurant window and stared at the young giant. "Gee," someone said, "Look at them paws." Robert didn't talk much while eating at the restaurant, but he lifted his little brother around like a "cigarette."

Robert finished his ham and eggs at the restaurant and the family departed in their seven-passenger sedan. "Robert loomed up in the back seat like an extra engine," an onlooker said.

Ralph McGhee was a Decatur friend of Wadlow's who was a salesman for a local shoe store. He met Robert through a shoe company representative. McGhee said Wadlow's shoes were actually size 36, not 39 as news items say. He said it cost the shoe company $500 just to make a pattern for the shoes, which McGhee estimated would have been 17 and 19 inches long and 8 to 9 inches wide.

Around the Metro St. Louis area, some children became frightened when they heard tales about the Alton giant. One was Carole Kesinger, of Carrollton, Ill., who was visiting with her parents' friend O.D. Poffenberger in Alton. Mrs. Poffenberger was taking care of her grandson as well as Kesinger. Mrs. Poffenberger's grandson was six years older than her and told tales of the "Alton giant" and how he would get you if you were out after dark in that area, typical tales for young boys who liked to frighten younger children.

After Mrs. Poffenberger's grandson left with some other kids, Kesinger wandered the streets looking for the Poffenberger house. A lady saw Kesinger wandering around alone and tried to help. She attempted to get information from Kesinger, but the little girl was just too terrified to tell her anything.

"She took me into her home and called the police to help me find my way back," Kesinger said. "I have often thought in later years of how I struggled with her to get out of the house before the police arrived. I was just too afraid to realize she was trying to help me. When the police arrived, they started driving around the neighborhood to see if I could recognize the house. As we were driving along, I saw my friend and the house almost at the same time."

Alton Patrolman Thomas Miller was called to investigate the Kesinger incident and after arriving drove only about two blocks with her when she said, "There's a boy I know." The boy was a neighborhood friend and in a few moments, Kesinger was back in the care of her grandmother.

Years later, Kesinger said she realized how kind and gentle Robert Wadlow was and couldn't imagine how she had been terrified by him.

"I often wished it could have been possible to meet this "Gentle Giant" and tell him how mistaken I was about him as a small child," Kesinger said.

Chapter 12

Death Of A Giant

The July 1940 evening before Robert Wadlow left Alton for the final time was typical for the family. The Wadlows had family and friends over before Robert and his father left in the morning for Manistee, Mich. Little did family and friends know it would be the final time they would see Alton's favorite son.

Bill Pitts was the last person outside the family in Alton to see Robert Wadlow before he made his last journey to Michigan. Pitts had a date with Helen Wadlow, one of Robert's sisters, the night before Robert left.

Pitts and Robert talked about politics, their favorite subject, that warm summer night at the Wadlow family home on Sanford Avenue. Pitts said Robert was happy and content. Robert looked as healthy as Pitts had seen him and in no way showed signs of the physical ailments to come.

"We were on the front porch conversing," Bill Pitts said. "I remember Robert's father, saying, 'Bob, you had better to go bed — we have to get up early tomorrow morning to go to Michigan.' Robert bid me good night. I watched him duck to get through the doorway. "

The first reports that Robert was having health problems came in the Alton Telegraph on July 6, 1940. The Telegraph headline read: "Robert Wadlow Ill in Hotel at Manistee, Mich."

The story said, "Robert Wadlow, Alton's young giant, is ill at a hotel in Manistee, Mich., where he has been laid up for three days. The malady is an infection of one of his feet, something similar to what caused him to be hospitalized in St. Louis at Barnes Hospital three years ago."

The infection was caused by a blister that had been noticed before he left Alton, but there was little concern, because Robert didn't normally have to stay on his feet much while traveling. A brace worn on his ankle chafed and the infection set in once they arrived in Manistee.

Robert had walked a long distance prior to the Manistee parade, further irritating the blister. He became extremely ill from the infection and had to sit in a car for several hours with his father during the crowded event. As soon as the streets cleared, he was rushed where he could receive medical attention.

Robert had received treatment at Barnes Hospital in St. Louis for infections and broken bones five times between 1930 and 1940. His father recognized the gravity of the infection this time and sent word that Addie should come and be with their son. Addie flew shortly thereafter into Muskegon, Mich., with their youngest son, Harold Jr., to be at her son's bedside.

The attending physician did not allow Robert to be moved from the hotel to a hospital because he thought they should move Robert as little as possible. Robert had been running a high fever, and his temperature soared because of the foot infection.

Harold Jr. vividly remembers the flight to Michigan. He was always excited to travel and see his big brother, but quickly after their arrival he knew something was not right.

"When we saw Robert in Michigan, he was very quiet," Harold Jr. recalled. "He had a very high temperature."

On July 8, 1940, the Alton Telegraph reported: "Robert Wadlow was reported making a satisfactory recovery from the foot infection that forced him to bed July 4 while he was participating in the Manistee National Forest Festival."

Nearly a week later on July 13, the Telegraph published a story headlined: "Robert Wadlow Runs 106-Degree Temperature."

The story said: "Robert Wadlow's condition is still 'slowly improving'" from a foot infection, the Associated Press reported. The inquiry was made after Helen Wadlow, Robert's sister, received word from her mother, Addie, that Robert had been running a temperature of 106 degrees."

Robert's condition continued to worsen on July 14, 1940, in the hotel. Harold Jr. remembers Robert continuing to be very quiet and the mood somber. During the day, physicians gave Robert a blood transfusion to help combat the infection and performed a minor operation on his foot during that evening. Robert's temperature remained 106 degrees all day. Doctors fed Robert through a tube.

Robert's final words at 10:30 the night of July 14, 1940, were "The doctor says I won't get home for the celebration."

Robert was referring to the golden wedding anniversary set for the last day of July for his grandfather and grandmother, who lived in Fort Lauderdale, Fla. Before Robert's illness, a celebration had been planned for the Wadlows at Harold Sr. and Addie's home in Alton. Robert had desperately wanted to attend and asked several times if he would be home in time for it, which the doctor told him he didn't think was possible.

Robert died peacefully at the age of 22 at 12:40 a.m., July 15, 1940, never recovering from the infection. Once Robert died, news flashed across the wire that the tallest man in modern history was gone.

Robert's hulking lifeless body was immediately taken to the Bradford Funeral Home in Manistee. One of the first problems for the Wadlow family was to find a casket that could hold their son. One of Harold Sr.'s brothers, Cecil E. Wadlow, was an undertaker in Lincoln, Neb. Cecil Wadlow recommended a metal casket built by the Grand Traverse Metal Casket Co. in Traverse City, Mich. The casket was 10 feet 6 inches long, 32 inches wide and 30 inches high, fitted in a redwood case made of 2-inch material. The coffin weighed almost 500 pounds, making it nearly 1,000 pounds that pallbearers would have to carry with Robert's 495-pound body.

"One of my uncles was an undertaker, and he and the others worked day and night to get the casket finished," Harold Jr. said.

Streeper Funeral Home in Alton was chosen to handle Robert's arrangements. Initially, the family favored a private funeral, but because Robert's life had been in the public eye so much, they didn't think it would be fair to keep the public from paying their respects as well. Robert Streeper, owner of Streeper Funeral Home, drove personally to Manistee to bring Robert's body home.

He was accompanied by Anthony Bellitto. The two arrived at the Streeper Funeral Home at 5:20 a.m., July 17, 1940, with the Wadlow body, after a 12-hour trip from Manistee.

It was decided because of the coffin's 1,000-pound weight, 16 pallbearers would be necessary, seven along each side of the coffin and one at each end. The funeral truck carrying the Wadlow coffin was backed from Main Street in Alton into the garage at the rear of the Streeper Funeral Home. The box containing the coffin was then placed on the garage floor and raised from its box by strap supports held by a crew of men.

From the garage, the coffin was carried along the driveway west of the building and around to the front porch. The wide double-door entrance was ample to admit the coffin, but the smaller door at the end of the main hallway leading into the chapel ante-room had to be enlarged. It was too narrow by some 6 inches.

A carpenter took care of the remodeling in the early morning hours but waited until after the coffin was positioned in the chapel before finishing the plastering and painting. A series of collapsible funeral carts had been welded together in advance to act as support for Robert's coffin.

On July 18, 1940, the City of Alton issued a statement to businesses to cease activity for five minutes on that day in tribute to Robert Wadlow. At 2 p.m. when funeral services began, a 5-minute memory period was set aside for Alton's most famous resident. The flag at Alton City Hall was to be flown at half-staff the day of the funeral until after funeral rites for Robert were concluded.

Robert Landiss was one of the DeMolays who took turns overseeing Robert's casket during the visitation at the funeral hours. One DeMolay stood at the head and another at the foot of the casket.

"People came in all day long," Landiss recalled. "Sometimes the lines were three blocks long outside. Some people who came were curious; others felt sorry for the family. I remember a lot of curiosity seekers being there."

Being one of the DeMolays guarding Robert's casket was an emotional experience for Landiss because of his familiarity with the Wadlow family.

"I was only a year younger than Robert, so it was sad for me," he said. "I remember that the family didn't stay by the casket the whole time. They did come out for certain people. There were so many strangers there that they couldn't have met everyone that came by. People came through day and night at the funeral home. People were there 24 hours a day for two days."

Lee Duncan was one of those who found it impossible to find his way into the funeral home. Duncan was working the evening shift, and when he got off work at midnight he decided to go by the funeral home to see Robert one last time.

"Bob Streeper decided to leave the funeral home open at night to accommodate all who wanted to view his remains,"

Duncan said. "After work the next evening I drove up to the corner of Washington Avenue and Brown Street before I saw the line of people waiting to get into the funeral home. They were two deep and stretched from the funeral home west on Edwards Street, then south on Washington Avenue and halfway down Brown Street toward Main, I got in line, and it was after 1 a.m. by the time I got into the funeral home. I don't remember too much as to how Robert looked, other than about normal. What struck me most was how big the casket was."

The Streeper Funeral Home carpet took such a beating from the thousands viewing Robert's body that it had to replace the carpeting after the funeral.

On July 18, groups began arriving at Streeper Funeral Home at 4 p.m., but a line did not start forming until 6 p.m. The peak was reached about 8:30 p.m. when the line extended from the front door of the funeral home on Edwards Street back to Main Street in Alton where it reached south two blocks past Main Street Methodist Church. People in the line stood about three or four to a row. Special traffic officers had been detailed to serve in the area of the funeral home, and there was a steady stream of cars with license plates from Missouri, Texas, North Dakota, South Dakota, New York and Louisiana.

Bob Lucker can still picture Robert Wadlow the last time anyone saw him in his casket at the funeral home. "I was one of thousands who came to pay their last respects," Lucker said. "I was struck by his gentle look. Alton had truly lost a remarkable young man."

The flow of callers was interrupted at 5 a.m., July 19, for a two-hour period for the family to have a few secluded moments with Robert. It was estimated that 27,000 people filed through Streeper Funeral Home before 10 a.m. on July 19. The number was determined by a count kept of the memorial leaflets handed to callers as they left the funeral home. Doors were reopened at 7 a.m. on July 19 for another throng of callers to come through. It had been planned to close the funeral home again at

10 a.m., but because of the intense traffic, it was later before visitation could be concluded.

The Oakwood Cemetery gates where Robert was to be buried were closed because the flow of cars in the cemetery was so great. Rumors circulated that the entire Wadlow family plot was to be fenced, but this rumor was unfounded.

Chapter 13

The Funeral Of Robert Wadlow

Hours before Robert Wadlow's burial at Oakwood Cemetery in Upper Alton, the undertakers' assistants and police had to open a pathway large enough for the coffin to be carried from the hearse to the grave. The morning crowd in the cemetery was estimated at 5,000.

It was estimated that between 10 a.m. Thursday and 1:45 p.m. Friday, 33,295 people visited Streeper Funeral Home in Alton. The number was determined by a mechanical checker held by an attendant. Before 10 a.m. Thursday, approximately 8,000 people visited the funeral home, making a total of 41,295 who viewed Robert Wadlow's body.

"There were thousands of people there," Harold Jr. said. "It was hard to understand so many being there, but things were so different then. People didn't have television or anything else. Robert was sort of like a movie star. I remember all those people down around the funeral home and cemetery. It was a mass of people. I had never seen anything like that before and never did after that."

When Jean Perry arrived for the funeral she saw car after car lined up near the funeral home. "The funeral process seemed more like a party than a funeral to me," Perry said.

The Rev. W.L. Hanbaum, pastor at Main Street Methodist Church, conducted the funeral service, assisted by the Rev. N.C. Henderson of Mt. Carmel, Ill., and the Rev. Otto Horsley of Herrin, Ill. The Masons conducted rites at Oakwood Cemetery. William F. Sinclair gave the oration; Forrest Cook was the chaplain; C.G. Smith was marshal and J.E. Juttemeyer was secretary.

Twelve Masons served as pallbearers during Robert's funeral. No eulogy was given during the funeral. Beginning at 1:30 p.m., Mrs. Alonzo Rosenberger, the funeral home organist, played the Robert Wadlow organ for 15 minutes in the Main Street Methodist Church over a public address system. Robert had told people about the organ throughout his travels and received nationwide contributions.

Rev. Hanbaum quoted Scripture during Wadlow's funeral from Apostle Paul's communication to Timothy referring to man's placing of his soul in God's trust for eternal life and quoted Bible assurances that "those who are in Him shall live forever."

The minister said that God's rule is paramount in the universe, as implied by Jesus Christ in the Garden of Gethesamane when the Savior said, "Not my will but Thine be done." Robert had an opportunity to serve the Lord and have great influences on the lives of others in only 22 years of living.

When the services concluded, there was a sudden surge of people outside seeking a close-up position to observe the pallbearers take the casket out of the funeral home and place it in the hearse to move to the cemetery. The pallbearers had difficulty moving through the throng of people to reach the hearse. The regular pallbearers had to have the assistance of six and sometimes eight people, to carry the weight of the casket and Robert's body. The hearse floor was given extra support of some planks to better distribute the weight.

When it came time to transport Robert Wadlow's body from

the funeral home to Oakwood Cemetery, the funeral directors had a problem — the casket would not fit in the hearse. The directors had to remove the end door of the hearse to fit Robert's enormous casket into it.

C. Travis Streeper, who later owned another Streeper Funeral Home on Washington Avenue in Alton from 1955-1984, assisted the directors at Robert's funeral by walking behind the hearse with the casket to the cemetery. The stretch to the cemetery was about a mile and a half. Robert's casket was tied into the hearse with a rope, said the late Travis' wife, Helen Streeper, also a classmate of Robert's at Alton High.

"My husband stayed behind the casket the entire way to the cemetery to make sure it was all right," Helen Streeper said. "It was sad. He was such a happy and well-liked person.

"The casket was huge," she said. "It was sad for my husband. Robert and Travis were both photographers and good friends. Robert didn't let being famous rub off on him. He was always just a person and himself."

James Schmitt was a DeMolay at the time of Robert's death, and he marched from Streeper Funeral Home to Oakwood Cemetery behind the hearse.

"I remember at the time, the funeral was nothing Alton had ever seen before," Schmitt said. "I remember we walked from Streeper Funeral Home to Oakwood Cemetery. There were probably 15 or 20 DeMolays behind the casket. I remember people crying along our way. This was so unexpected for Alton people. There were a lot of sad people at the funeral, but also a lot of curiosity seekers."

Robert's casket extended about 3 feet out of the hearse on its trek to Oakwood Cemetery. The hearse moved slowly up Main Street and eventually into Oakwood Cemetery.

Robert Landiss will never forget the walk from the funeral home to Oakwood Cemetery through Upper Alton. Along the way, the streets were lined with people wall to wall watching the hearse creep by.

"I remember it being very quiet as we walked behind the hearse to the cemetery," Landiss said. "It was a lifetime memory. There were people everywhere. There was less of a crowd at the cemetery, although a lot of people did go to the cemetery. Some went, but stood somewhat from the activities."

Once Robert's body entered Oakwood Cemetery, a Masonic ritual service order for the dead was performed by William F. Sinclair. He had been an instructor of Robert's at the Franklin Masonic Lodge and described Robert as one of the most brilliant pupils he had ever known.

When the service was over, most of the crowd retired. Then the casket was lowered into a concrete vault that was at the bottom of the grave and enclosed in a red cedar box. The cedar box lid was lowered to cover it, then a concrete mixer was rolled up and started preparing material to seal the casket with steel. Guards patrolled Robert's grave after the funeral for a week. The Wadlow family feared people would take flowers as souvenirs from the grave.

Telegraph photographer Robert Graul was on hand when Robert's pallbearers positioned the 1,000-pound casket in the wooden box that had been shipped by the manufacturer enclosed in a concrete vault.

"They had the concrete mixer right on the grounds of Oakwood Cemetery," Graul said. "I saw the concrete being poured in the vault. The concrete was a good idea; there was some talk of the body being stolen for scientific reasons. The Wadlow family was determined to prevent something like that from happening. But they didn't allow for the extra depth of the casket, which is why the ground in Robert's cemetery plot is about a foot higher than any of the other plots."

The family remained at the site until the concrete was poured, which ensured no one would be able to dig up his body for experimentation. The reason Robert Wadlow was buried in concrete was due in part because of mistrust associated with the libel suits and nationwide fascination with the world's tallest man. The Wadlow family simply wanted peace and quiet for their son after he died.

"All my family wanted when he died was for people to leave him alone," Harold Jr. said. "The doctor who analyzed him in St. Louis was a nasty person. My family worried he would find a way to have Robert's body dug up. We believed he wanted to experiment on him. He was the reason they had the vault put in and concrete poured in the ground. There couldn't be someone out at the cemetery at night watching the grave."

Soon after Robert's funeral, the Wadlow family retreated to the family home on Sanford Avenue and proceeded to burn many of Robert's clothes and much of his furniture. Harold Jr. said the family burned the materials because they didn't want them to get into the wrong hands. Harold Sr. and Addie Wadlow were afraid that future generations would attempt to portray Robert as a "freak," which the family spent his whole life trying to prevent from happening.

The family, especially Addie, yearned for the publicity and talk about Robert to go away. "They wanted Robert to be able to rest in peace," Harold Jr. said. "Mother understood people were curious and he was in the limelight, but she couldn't bear it. When he died, mother burned most of his clothes and many of his other items. Mother was a very kind and wonderful person but was private and couldn't deal with all the publicity."

A couple of times a week, Harold Sr. and Addie Wadlow drove to the cemetery and somberly remembered their oldest son.

"Mother used to come out all the time and put flowers around Robert's grave," Harold Jr. said. "Dad was always cutting crab grass out here. They made it look nice and always remembered him."

Chapter 14

A Photographer's Favorite Subject

Robert K. Graul shot nearly 80 percent of the 100 Robert Wadlow photos still in existence, over a four-year period beginning on Jan. 15, 1936, and ending with Robert's funeral on July 19, 1940.

On Jan. 15, 1936, Graul, 22, began working as a professional photographer for the Alton Evening Telegraph. Graul's first photo assignment was for a 100th anniversary section of the Telegraph, taking a shot of the senior class party at the YWCA in Alton. In the senior class photo that day was 8-foot-4 Alton High student Robert Wadlow.

"I was more or less unaccustomed to the new Speed Graphic camera I was using with a huge flashbulb," Graul said. "It was the size of a 100-watt bulb today in those days. The students were assembled in the lobby of the YWCA, and I stood on a table across the room with a camera. We did not have a wide angle lens at that time. I shot two shots, enough to capture both ends of the group. I was nervous. I didn't have much training."

Graul had spent the previous year working at the Kopp

Studio in Alton taking portraits, after graduating from Shurtleff College in Alton with a chemistry degree. Before that shoot at the YWCA, Graul had never heard of the world's tallest man.

"Robert's name was never mentioned at Shurtleff College around me," Graul said.

On the day of Graul's first professional photo, Wadlow was 18. He was in the back of the group that day, and Graul did not speak with him.

"I was amazed at how tall he was," Graul said. "He was as tall as the room. He stood under an arch formed by two wooden columns, leading to the entrance to the swimming pool and the gym."

Later, the high school photo became a permanent piece of Alton's history. It showed how tall Robert was in relation to the rest of his class. Graul photographed Robert again a week or so later at the Wadlow family home on Brown Street. On that day, Graul snapped pictures of Robert and Harold Jr. together with their siblings.

"Robert was affable and willing to pose or sit anywhere I asked him to," Graul said. Graul immediately noticed a strong bond between Robert and Harold Jr.

"He was very loving toward his brother. I could tell he loved him deeply. Robert was proud of his baby brother. If Harold Jr. was out of view when I was taking a picture, he'd ask his brother to come and be with him. He picked Harold up and sat him on his lap."

"A lot of times older and younger brothers experience animosity toward each other, but that didn't exist between Robert and Harold Jr.," Graul said. "When I went to the family home there was constant, happy interaction."

Photography was not easy in the mid-1930s. Photographers didn't shoot in the machine gun style of today, which is the reason there are so few photographs of Robert Wadlow. Not many photos were taken of the world's tallest man during his lifetime, except by family and friends.

"I photographed Robert mostly on his birthdays," Graul said. "My partner, Leland Heppner, shot him on some of his birthdays. I shot him at special events, like when he got his Masonic ring. Robert studied hard with his trainer to be a Mason. He was very elated when he became a Mason."

Robert received his Masonic ring at Goulding's jewelry store on Third Street in Alton. The store owner Robert Goulding presented the ring to Robert.

"Robert was somber at the Masonic ring presentation," Graul said. "A representative of the jewelry company that made the ring was there, too. I had a little bit of awe when I took his picture. We didn't make a whole lot of him being the tallest man in the world at that time. He was just a tall person."

Graul was glad Robert got to travel as much as he did with his father. Robert traveled to every state in the United States. When Robert died, it left a lasting impact on young Graul that he carried through all his years. "I was very, very sad when he died. You never know how long a person like him is going to live, so I guess it wasn't a great surprise when he died."

Graul remembers Robert's funeral well, even six decades later.

"It was an amazing number of people who turned out to view the body at the funeral home in Alton," Graul said. "I shot a photograph when the casket was closed and two DeMolays were standing by as guards. You always tingle when you shoot someone who is in a casket. I guess that was one of my hardest shots because I knew him so well. The crowd of people is what I remember the most."

Graul didn't recall too many sobbing spectators around the funeral home when he was in attendance. Most were curious, he said, simply interested in Robert. "You might say some loved him, some were nothing but curious," Graul said.

He said he knew the funeral proceedings were extremely difficult for Harold and Addie Wadlow, but especially his mother.

"She was adverse to publicity," Graul said. "There was hardly anything in the paper from the time he was born until the time of his death with the exception of about four years when I started photographing him. Previous to that, you couldn't find a picture of Robert. Addie protected Robert very much. I'm glad the Wadlow legend lives on thanks to that time period."

Graul is thankful to be a part of the Robert Wadlow legacy, although he doesn't feel any great responsibility about it.

"I'm happy people all over the world get to see my work," he said. "It was just in the line of my job, that's all. I'm glad I could do it. The popularity of Robert Wadlow has changed with the times. For Alton people, Robert was an ordinary, tall boy, nothing extraordinary. For people away from Alton, he was incredible."

Graul said many people around Alton seem to have a favorite story about the giant that they pass through generations.

"Robert is Alton's favorite son," Graul said. "Robert's fame spread all over the world because there never has been anybody else like him. He was just a kind and gentle fellow. I think he was outstanding because of his size and gentlemanly nature."

"Harold Jr. always accepted his big brother, Robert," Graul said. "He was always in sight of his big brother when I was around, and always wanted to be in every photo with his big brother. Harold was always very cognizant that his brother was unique."

Sometimes today when he is out on a pleasant day shooting, Graul's thoughts turn back in time to the 1930s and 1940 when he chronicled Robert Wadlow's life with his photographs.

"It was always a special occasion when I got the chance to take Robert's photo," Graul said. "It was quite an experience sitting in the family home and being welcome even though we are more or less in a forum that was prying. I guess that is most of what a newspaper does — looks into people's lives."

Graul will never forget his first photograph in 1936 of Robert Wadlow and the Alton High senior class. It's hard to think of a more dramatic way to have started a newspaper career that spanned more than 40 years.

Chapter 15

Preserving The Wadlow Legend

The Alton Museum of History and Art is nestled among shade trees across the street from the Robert Wadlow Statue on the campus of Southern Illinois University Edwardsville School of Dental Medicine in Loomis Hall. The structure is a brick, Federal style building with a Greek classical front entrance. Loomis Hall was built in 1832 and is listed as a significant building within Upper Alton's Historic District and is on the National Register of Historic Places.

Harold Jr. loved the museum exhibit for his brother. He said any time he visited the museum he had wonderful feelings about the past and his family heritage. He wished more of Robert's artifacts could have been preserved.

"Mother got rid of his things over the years," Harold Jr. said during the summer of 2000. "She was a very private person and was very protective of Robert and Robert's memory. Once he died, she wanted to forget; she wanted everybody to drop it."

Charlene Gill, one of the founders of the Alton Museum and the president emeritus, respected Addie Wadlow's feelings about protecting Robert's memory. Gill's sister-in-law spoke with Addie and was aware of her feelings about having any type of exhibit. The museum respected her wishes and did not open a Wadlow exhibit until after her death.

Without Harold Jr.'s contributions, the Robert Wadlow exhibit would not have been possible. He personally donated Robert's eyeglasses, a copy of his Masonic ring, Robert's personal Bible, wallet, a handkerchief box and even his brother's tennis racket.

Graul watched the Wadlow display grow from the beginning. "We also didn't make any emphasis on Robert Wadlow until we had space," he said. "I feel I contributed something to the display with my photographs. I'm glad we preserved Robert's life."

Harold Jr. lived in St. Louis when the Alton museum opened its doors in 1971. Gill was one of the people guiding the museum board from its beginnings.

"We didn't know Harold Jr. until he moved back to Alton after his retirement," she said. "He came to visit us at the museum then."

Gill was born in Alton in 1924 and had actually met Robert in 1936 in nearby Brighton, Ill. Gill was in the sixth grade when she met Robert at the Brighton Village Hall. Robert spoke between acts at a senior class play while they changed the sets behind the curtains. The children could barely contain their excitement the night Robert spoke.

"When the curtains came down, Robert Wadlow came out in front and people gave him an ovation," Gill said. "He was taking elocution lessons from Mrs. Lancaster in Alton and practicing the art of public speaking. Wc all lined up to shake his hand. I remember looking up and up and up to see his face."

For weeks, Gill and her friends talked about seeing Alton's Gentleman Giant. Gill and other museum board members have always remained steadfast in protecting the integrity of Robert Wadlow's memory with their exhibit and tours.

"We all cherish the memory of Robert and are pleased that we developed the exhibit on him," Gill said. "We always wanted it to be in good taste. Robert Graul is responsible for the actual photography. Robert Graul and Norma Miller had the idea of enlarging the photograph of Robert receiving his Masonic ring from jeweler Robert Goulding, gluing the photo to plywood, and cutting it out so it is free standing. There is now a Robert Wadlow likeness of the correct scale. Many copies have been made locally so that people can compare their size with that of Robert."

The museum also has a huge sled that Robert once rode up and down Milton neighborhood hills during his childhood. A camera believed to be used when Robert was a member of the Camera Club at Alton High is also in the museum collection. In addition to his Bible and glasses are a pen and knife of Robert's in a glass case. Robert's graduation cap and gown were donated by the company that made them after a request was made from the museum. One of Robert's size 37 well-worn shoes was also donated. The Optimist Club in Alton donated money for a glass case to hold and protect Robert's cherished items.

In 1971, Charles "Tim" Leone made a documentary titled, "The Story of Robert," which has been shown nationwide and abroad. The film is available for tourists to see when they visit the museum.

Leone became acquainted with the Alton giant while researching a film about the 1930s outlaws Bonnie and Clyde.

Peggy Leone is proud of her husband's documentary about Robert Wadlow. She said "The Story of Robert" has been shown on television stations all over the United States and is now even being played in countries around the world, including Israel and Russia.

"The movie is being translated to Russian, Arabic and Hebrew," Leone added. "The movie is too good to just sit around on a shelf."

Andrew Gordon Sr. came from London to the Alton museum because his son, Andrew Gordon Jr., 13, had read about Robert Wadlow in the Guinness Book of World Records. Andrew

Gordon Sr., his wife, Anne, and their sons, Andrew Jr. and Simon visited the Robert Wadlow displays.

"It's absolutely a brilliant site," Andrew Gordon Sr. said of the museum's Wadlow display. "It is well laid out and well explained. We all compared our heights. I came up to his elbows, and I'm 5-foot-9. It was an amazing thing to look up and up and up at the top of his head."

Nicholas Brats, 18, of Toulouse, France, visited the museum on his trip to America and described the museum as a blast to the past. He planned to return to France and communicate his impressions. "Maybe the pictures will explain everything to my friends," he said. "It's an amazing story. I first saw it in the Guinness Book of Records."

Greg Hind and Glen Reither, members of the famous Little River Band of Melbourne, Australia, also were Robert Wadlow exhibit visitors. Hind described Robert Wadlow's story as "mind-boggling." "I can't believe there is as much information around about him," he said. "The footage in the video and photos are great shots. I tried to walk the streets of Alton while I was here and picture what it was like to have been around during his time."

Reither thought the "The Story of Robert" video was first-class, and he also fell in love with the Alton museum. "The museum is cool," Reither said. "There are not a lot of things like this throughout the world. I think it's a great tribute to Robert."

It's not uncommon any day of the week to find a person in the museum's Wadlow exhibit from any foreign country. When they leave, because of the exhibit, they have a clear impression of what it was like to have been the tallest man in the world in a small, Midwestern river town.

Chapter 16

The Wadlow Statue

When Steve Tassinari came up with the idea to build a statue for Robert Wadlow in the early 1980s, Alton, Ill., was facing a decline. Alton had lost the Owens-Illinois glass plant in 1983 and with it about 2,000 jobs. Amoco Refinery and Shell Refinery were also trimming back in Wood River, and the steel industry was experiencing a downward trend, affecting employment at Alton's Laclede Steel and nearby Granite City Steel. Unemployment had risen to 10 percent in Alton.

Tassinari had been like most Alton area boys and had placed his young body beside Robert Wadlow's grave in Oakwood Cemetery in Upper Alton to gauge his height against Robert's. Tassinari got interested in Robert again in the early 1980s when he was showing his son how tall Wadlow was with a yardstick over his head. He watched Tim Leone's video "The Story of Robert" and suddenly was motivated to establish a permanent monument for the world's tallest man.

He felt the Alton community needed to start building the town's spirit back, rather than tearing anything down. Tassinari, then a sales executive with the Xerox Corporation in St. Louis, co-chaired the Robert Wadlow Statue drive with Ron Vanata, a vice president of marketing for the 7-Up Co. in St. Louis.

A statue commission was formed and met weekly on Fridays for three years at the Alton Telegraph to discuss and plan the project. Telegraph Publisher Steve Cousley served as host, and one of the integral reasons the statue project was successful was his ability to unify the commission members and the community through the newspaper's editorials.

Tassinari said the commission's goal was to preserve the memory of Robert Wadlow. The commission recognized that Robert was a gentle, strong-willed man and an important part of the history and culture of Alton. He was a native and inspiration to both young and old. The commission told contributors that it was not his great size, but his undaunted spirit, humor and gentle demeanor in the face of his handicap that made him worthy of remembrance.

Tassinari felt it was a big risk when he first went public with his idea about the statue, but in the end there was a lot of fulfillment.

"We did a very bold thing," Tassinari said. "There were no rules. We could have been tarred and feathered and laughed out of town. There was lot of potential embarrassment, but we did it, and the key to the success was a very unselfish group. I had worked for Xerox and applied some of my training to the project. I was young and fearless at the time."

When the campaign got under way, Tassinari and the group raised $10,000 from Alton-Godfrey Rotary and Alton area Optimist clubs. The commission had enough money to pay an artist at that point.

The Rotary and Optimist clubs announced their commitment to the project on Aug. 17, 1984. The following month, a joint meeting was held to announce that native Altonian Ned Giberson had been commissioned to sculpt the statue. In November 1984, the commission fund passed the $33,000 mark after 1,200 telephone calls and the sale of thousands of Robert Wadlow buttons.

In December 1984, the Junior League in Alton donated $10,000 to the Robert Wadlow Statue project. The Olin Corp. in East Alton donated 3,000 pounds of copper alloy for the statue in December 1984. The 3,000 pounds of copper alloy metal had a commercial value of approximately $2,000 at the time. The commission had $50,000 at this point in the fund-raising drive.

Area school children helped sell buttons for the Wadlow Statue project. The Alton museum designed a bank in the shape of Robert's shoe that made a tour of schools to allow children to donate funds. Pupils gave their nickels and dimes to the bank. In January 1985, the Alton Board of Realtors pledged $5,000 for the Wadlow project and helped it come closer to the commission's goal of $53,450. Written statue site offers came from Alton Square, Upper Alton Cemetery, Washington Square, Franklin Masonic Lodge and the Visitor Center in Downtown Alton. A site at Southern Illinois University School of Dental Medicine (formerly Shurtleff College) was also suggested and eventually chosen. Guidelines for site selection were set Oct. 6, 1984, and the university board committee approved the official site in June 1985.

Giberson began work on the actual statue with three 28-inch mockups in January 1985. In April 1985, he finished the 9-foot clay model. In June 1985, latex rubber molds were applied to the clay model and plaster "positives" were cast from the latex models, then transported to the Johnson Atelier Technical Institute of Sculpture in Mercerville, N.J., where it was cast into bronze. In the end, the committee raised more than $70,000 and the final cost was $73,000.

"There really wasn't a formula for the success of the project," Tassinari said. "It was a challenge. It was something we had to do from the heart. Robert Wadlow is fascinating. He is the claim to fame to a lot of the older folks in Alton. He literally outgrew society."

Giberson, an Alton native and a young, aspiring artist, was a graduate of Guilford College in Greensboro, N.C., with a master's of fine arts with concentration in sculpture from Southern Illinois University at Edwardsville. Giberson, like many from Alton, also grew up hearing tales about Robert Wadlow.

"My father, Dudley Giberson, knew Robert," Giberson said. "I've always been interested in him. It was my first monumental sculpture, and being the world's tallest person made it even bigger. Life-size sculptures are typically 6 feet, and this one was 9 feet. It was overwhelming in some ways, but I had a feeling I could do it."

The sculpture took 13 months for Giberson to complete. The young artist poured over hundreds of Wadlow photos and read everything he possibly could about him. Giberson said all his Wadlow maquettes were fairly similar. "In one, his hands were in his pocket; another was one with him holding his hip; and another grasping a cane," Giberson said. "The hip shot was my favorite; I thought it was a natural pose. I always do a lot of research before I begin a sculpture. I work toward getting the essence of an individual and it's all about understanding them."

Giberson and the Robert Wadlow Statue Commission were in unison on the project. The young artist attempted to be respectful of the Alton community in the Robert Wadlow piece. Giberson wanted to hear what the community had to say about the project, and he kept his studio open one day a week so people could comment and share their experiences about Robert. Giberson listened to everyone who came into his studio. Many of the old-timers came to the studio and spent hours sharing their stories about Robert.

The "Wadlowfest," a celebration to dedicate the statue, was held Oct. 19-20, 1985, in Upper Alton. On Saturday, Oct. 19, booths were set up on Main Street that included Jerome Hagen and Harold Kirsch, who traveled with Wadlow, classmates and Harold Jr. "The Story of Robert," Tim Leone's film, was also shown at the Cameo Theater several times that day. Giberson made a slide presentation on the making of the statue.

On Sunday, Oct. 20, the "Wadlowfest" continued with booths, music groups and the statue's unveiling. More than 2,500 people attended the day the statue was unveiled.

"Robert Wadlow is with us again," Tassinari told the throng of people who wore coats on the cool, damp October afternoon. "Wadlow was the champion of humanity, especially for the handicapped."

A highlight of the program was an original Wadlow song by the Gilson Brown School chorus of Alton, directed by Mary Kay Mosby. "I want to stand tall like Robert Wadlow," sang the children. "I want to be the best I can be and make the best of me." Mosby wrote six to eight songs to tell the story about Robert's life so children could identify with him.

"I wanted children to know that in spite of his physical problems he tried to be the best he could be," Mosby said. "For many, life isn't fair. There was a lot of television coverage and the kids got to see themselves on TV the day the statue was dedicated."

At the conclusion of the formal program, television film crews were ready and camera shutters clicked as the wooden cover was lifted, showing the bronze likeness of Wadlow. The statue of Wadlow's familiar figure, wearing his wire-rimmed glasses, stands tall under the trees on the campus of Southern Illinois University Edwardsville School of Dental Medicine.

Spectators broke out in cheers and applauded. "Wow, he was a big man! It's beautiful. It's great." Harold Wadlow Jr. remembered that the day was one of the best days of his life. "People came from across the world for the dedication," Harold Jr. said. "It was very special."

The White House sent a telegram to the Oct. 15, 1985, gathering in Alton. President Ronald Reagan said: "I am pleased to send greetings to all those gathered for the dedication of a statue of Robert Pershing Wadlow at Southern Illinois University in Alton, Illinois. I remember the sensation that Robert Wadlow caused in the late '30s. He was truly a 'Gentle Giant,' a kind and good-humored man who died at a tragically young age. I commend the organizations and individuals that have contributed to the erection of this statue commemorating him. I send you my best wishes. God bless you."

The Robert Wadlow Statue today attracts tourists to Alton from all over the world. The Alton Museum guest registry has signatures from every U.S. state, Australia, Japan, Canada, the Philippines, Indonesia, England, Germany and Ireland. Each week, tourists from around the world visit the statue and the museum.

"Part of this is the Alton story about Robert, too," Gill said. "The people of Alton had a spirit of acceptance of Robert's frailty and loved him for who he was. To others throughout the world, Robert Wadlow showed people who are challenged in some fashion that it is possible to move beyond frailty."

Henry B. Lenhardt, now deceased, remembered the 1936 Alton High School class having a reunion the summer following the 1985 commemoration. They assembled at the Wadlow Statue where a wreath was placed in memory of their largest and most famous classmate. Lenhardt, the tallest in the 1936 class at 6-foot-4, was selected to speak in a syndicated television talk-show interview with Sally Jessy Raphael. "Being only two feet shorter than the tallest graduate has always been my claim to fame," Lenhardt said.

Robert Graul was part of the Wadlow Statue process from the beginning, serving on the statue committee to select the site and the artist, Ned Giberson.

"It's a beautiful statue," Graul said. "I love the statue; I think it is great, certainly a tribute to Ned Giberson the sculptor. I was very happy when it was unveiled and glad to have made a lasting memorial to Robert."

Robert Fleming must have been another attracted to Robert Wadlow's ability to move beyond his disabilities. In 2000, thanks to the efforts of Fleming, a local community activist for the disabled, the Robert Wadlow Statue area now has curb cuts, and anyone with any disability can wheel to see the world's tallest man. Fleming died at age 48 on May 5, 1998, losing a battle from a fourth brain tumor. Robert Wadlow inspired Fleming with his ability to love everyone around him, even if they poked fun at him. Fleming spent $300 out of his own pocket for a curb cut in January 1989.

Today, an estimated 100,000 people a year stop and see the statue. Giberson realizes the impact the Robert Wadlow piece has had on society.

"I captured a folk hero," Giberson said. "There is no doubt about it, the Wadlow piece changed my life. I'm overwhelmed at the response we have had through the years."

Tassinari believes the key to the statue commission's success was the early recognition that Robert Wadlow was not just a tall boy, but a fellow who overcame a severe handicap. "He was also a gentleman and had a kind heart," Tassinari said. "The statue means a lot to me today. A lot of people come to visit this old river town to see his statue. This is one of the ways this town renewed itself."

The statue serves as a memory and testament to the giant and a continued renewal of Alton, which was once a great Midwestern river city.

Chapter 17

Wadlow An International Sensation

An appearance on the daytime Oprah Winfrey show is one of the most coveted spots in American television. In 1996, Oprah Winfrey did a segment on town oddities and featured Robert Wadlow. The Alton Museum's Charlene Gill made a personal appearance in Chicago on Oprah's show and carried one of Robert's shoes. Winfrey stood next to a life-size cutout of the world's tallest man, which dwarfed her, and talked of how Robert Wadlow was born and lived in Alton, Ill. The day after the Oprah Winfrey show, a person in Indiana contacted the Alton Museum of History & Art and donated the match to the Wadlow shoe seen on the show.

The Robert Wadlow Web site (www.altonweb.com/history/wadlow) today is one of the most visited in the world. Designed by Alan McHugh, it was unveiled in January 1996. Since that time it has had more than 500,000 visitors. In March 1998, the Wadlow Web site was one of the Yahoo Picks of the Week.

The Wadlow Web site went on to be one of the Yahoo Picks of the Year and was voted fourth out of 52 top weekly Picks for the Year in 1998. The Web sites were judged on interesting information, story and design. Hundreds of people have also responded to a message board on the Robert Wadlow Web site. Many of them saw Robert during his journeys across the country.

McHugh arrived on the scene in Alton in 1987 and had been fascinated by the Wadlow Statue, the Alton Museum of History & Art and Wadlow's story. Charlene Gill's appearance on the Oprah Winfrey Show was an extra incentive to get the Web site going. "Obviously, this was a labor of love for me," McHugh said. "The site has remained unchanged since mid-1996 except for some updates. The Robert Wadlow story is a slice of Americana. Robert Wadlow is a folk hero, a unique individual who lived a unique life."

Millie Bentley recalls traveling in London later in the 1990s after seeing Wadlow in the 1930s and seeing an extraordinary sight. While traveling on a street car, she saw a poster of Robert Wadlow looming above other posters in a store window.

"I laughed and said what a small world it is after all," Bentley said. "I couldn't believe it. It took me back to seeing him in Cape Girardeau, Mo., many years earlier."

On Aug. 18, 1998, Wadlow's life took center stage on "Guinness World Records: Primetime" on the national Fox network. The taping featured interviews with Harold Jr. and footage at the museum. In late December 1999, "Ripley's Believe It Or Not" television series did a taping for the TBS Network in Alton about Robert Wadlow.

In May 2000, the British Broadcasting Company came to Alton to shoot footage on Wadlow. The BBC was taping for a segment on the Discovery Channel, which aired in the fall of 2000. Each week, the Alton Museum of History & Art ships Robert Wadlow packages throughout the world with videos, clippings and photographs.

Robert Wadlow's birthdays were always a special time in his life. Every year during his life, the Wadlow family had a large birthday party with cake and candles.

After the Alton Museum opened its Robert Wadlow section, it annually hosted a birthday display in commemoration of Robert's birthday. Each year, Duke's Bakery in Alton has donated a cake and candles. Each year, the remaining Wadlow family members are invited to attend the party. Harold Jr. often attended, helped light the candles on the cake and had a piece of cake in remembrance of his legendary big brother. Schoolchildren in Alton are invited to attend the birthday party each year.

Robert Wadlow's 80th birthday celebration Feb. 20-22, 1998, was the biggest Gentle Giant birthday fete ever in Alton. The world's tallest woman — Sandy Allen — 7-feet-7-inches and 400 pounds, visited Alton. At the time, Allen was 44. Originally from Chicago, she was listed in the Guinness Book of World Records as the tallest living woman. Allen was excited about coming to Alton to celebrate Robert Wadlow's birthday in his hometown.

"I never met Robert Wadlow, but I feel a kinship with him because of our height," Allen said. "I understand how he felt when people stared at him just because he stood out in a crowd."

Doctors discovered a similar affliction in Allen that Robert possessed. She had a tumor in her pituitary gland that was removed when she was 14 years old. Allen was 7 feet tall at age 14.

Robert Wadlow's 80th birthday celebration was the most spectacular, Gill said. "The children love the birthday celebration every year," she explained. "We show Tim Leone's film and adjourn to the Pioneer Room for birthday cake. We plan to have the birthday celebration as long as we can."

Harold Jr. enjoyed meeting Sandy Allen.

"Sandy Allen was a nice person," he said. "She did a nice job while she was here in Alton."

Harold Jr. was joined by his niece, Barbara Upchurch, and her son, Robert, 9, of Bonaqua, Tenn., for Robert's 80th birthday festivities.

Mary Kay Mosby's Alton schoolchildren again performed "Stand Tall Kids" for the birthday event. Personal letters of remembrances of Wadlow from his friends were also on display, along with other Wadlow memorabilia.

Mary Ann Warmack, Alton Museum coordinator during the celebration, thought Robert set a solid example for people with disabilities.

"Robert Wadlow overcame a lot in his life," Warmack said. "Sandy Allen was a fantastic lady and fun to be around during the 80th birthday. She had a good sense of humor. This celebration showed people what Robert meant to Alton."

The birthday celebration was Gill's idea because she wanted to make everyone aware of what kind of person Robert Wadlow was and what he meant to the Alton area and the fact that he was the area's greatest goodwill ambassador.

The Franklin Lodge No. 25 Masonic Lodge at 1513 Washington Ave. in Alton is another place that has always protected and preserved the memory of Robert.

Today there is a Robert Wadlow Room at Franklin Lodge. The room contains Wadlow booklets and clippings galore; one of his trademark shoes, a replica of the Mason ring, his favorite family chair and the registry from the funeral home for his time there. The room was started at the Masonic Lodge shortly after Robert's death.

The Wadlow chair was specially built by the Galax Furniture Company in Galax, Va., to hold Robert's nearly 500-pound body. The chair weighs approximately 450 pounds. The covering and style of chair was selected by Robert himself from one of the regular numbers carried in stock by the furniture company.

In the Franklin Lodge Wadlow Room, a person can press a button and hear Robert's voice in a New York City interview in 1939. When Harold Sr. died in 1940, the Masonic Lodge received the copy of Robert's Masonic ring for the Wadlow

Room. The copy of the ring was made through Goulding's Jewelry. Over the years, people have contributed other items for the room. Robert Wadlow is one of the world's best known Masons.

Cecil Griesbaum, a 33rd-degree Scottish Mason and Franklin Lodge secretary for 33 years from 1959 to 1992, is 89 now and has been a Mason since 1947. "I was a little older than him; I am 89 now," he said. "I have been a Mason since 1947. It's an amazing story. I think we have done a good job preserving his memory."

Robert Landiss often shows people how big Wadlow's foot was on the steps going up to the Wadlow Room and how he had to walk to get upstairs. He explains to people how he had to shuffle from side to side to go up and down stairs. "People can't believe it," Landiss said of how hard it was for Robert to take the size 37 shoe, which weighed four pounds and was 19 inches long, up and down to travel steps.

Hundreds have strolled through the Wadlow Room at the Masonic Lodge over the years. The room has also been a place for Mason members who knew Robert Wadlow to share stories with sons and daughters. Landiss and the other Masonic Lodge members said the Wadlow Room would be there for future generations to witness the facts and artifacts of the world's tallest person.

The Masons have worked hard to preserve Wadlow's memory and explain how he was a gentle, kind person.

"I think it's important to know his family didn't want to make a circus freak out of him," Earl Griesbaum said. "He wasn't that kind of a person. He was an ordinary person; he was just big."

Jim Siatos, a Franklin Masonic Lodge member for 20 years, has worked to help preserve Wadlow's memory at the Washington Avenue location in Alton. Siatos is in hopes the lodge can laminate the newspapers and other papers in the near future.

"The real Masonic ring is put away," Harold Jr. said during

the summer 2000. "The one at the Masonic Lodge is a dupli-
cate."

Robert Wadlow never played golf, but the Alton City
Council agreed to rename Municipal Golf Course at Golf Road
and Homer Adams Parkway after the world's tallest man during
the 80th birthday celebration. The name was the idea of the late
George Spence of Alton. The measure won with a 7-0 vote.

Alton Mayor Don Sandidge and City Council realized Robert
Wadlow was never Jack Nicklaus but thought the decision to
name a golf course was another way to honor Alton's most
famous citizen ever.

Chapter 18

Wadlow, Medical Analysis

D r. Philip Cryer, a Washington University physician and doctor of internal medicine, has a theory that a tumor in Robert Wadlow's pituitary gland caused his abnormal growth. Cryer, 60, a faculty member since 1971, is the Washington University director of the division of endocrinology, diabetes and metabolism.

The pituitary gland produces the growth hormone in the human body. The two problems with tumors in the pituitary gland are giantism, which normally occurs in childhood, and acromegaly, typically found in adulthood.

Giantism is the excessive development of the body or a body part. It is an abnormal condition characterized by excessive size and stature, caused most frequently by an over secretion of growth hormone. Giantism associated with normal body proportions and normal sexual development usually results from over secretion of growth hormone in early childhood.

Acromegaly, a disease caused by excessive secretion of growth hormone from the pituitary gland in adult life, is manifested by headaches and enlargement of the hands, feet and jaw.

"I think Robert Wadlow almost assuredly had a tumor in his pituitary gland," Dr. Cryer said. "If the surgery doesn't work to correct the pituitary gland problems today, medication is then given. There has been a lot of progress made since Robert Wadlow was alive. Great progress was made in the field of endocrinology regarding pituitary gland surgery in the 1960s, which was one big step forward, then in the last 20 years medication that depresses the growth hormone. I would hope what happened to Robert would not happen today."

The pituitary gland is a pea-sized, small vascular endocrine gland at the base of the brain and found in most vertebrates. It consists of an anterior and posterior lobe. The posterior lobe secretes hormones affecting renal functions and contraction of smooth muscle reproduction. The anterior lobe secretes hormones that control and regulate most of the other endocrine glands. Thus, this gland directly or indirectly controls and regulates most basic body functions.

Most of Cryer's patients have acromegaly. A pituitary gland tumor today is surgically removed. The surgery is tedious and delicate, but the survival rate is high. Today, two-thirds to three-fourths of those who have pituitary gland surgery are cured.

One problem with excessive growth is that a person doesn't go through puberty. With acromegaly, the length of a person's lifespan doesn't differ that much from a normal person.

Dr. Cryer was uncertain how long Robert would have lived without the foot infection. He thought it was unlikely he would have lived to old age because of his pituitary gland problems. If Robert had been born today, Dr. Cryer is certain he and his colleagues at Washington University could have cured him of his growth problems with either corrective surgery or medication.

"Robert would probably have been tall, but not nearly as tall," Dr. Cryer said. "Today, we are put on this type of medical problem early in a person's life."

Dr. Cyril MacBryde, who studied Robert Wadlow in the Barnes Hospital Metabolism Ward in St. Louis, saw Robert from the time he was 10 1/2 years old to 18 days before his death. MacBryde was on hand for Robert's last examination

June 27, 1940, when he was measured at 8 feet 11.1 inches and weighed 491 pounds.

"The height measurement alone does not convey properly the impression of the immense size one perceived in the presence of this large human being," the doctor said in a narrative. "Let us say that he was almost 9 feet tall and compare him with a taller than average man who is 6 feet tall. This would be an excess of 50 percent above the other man's height. Robert was lean and never the least bit fat or overweight. At age 21, Robert weighed 491 pounds. He was almost three times the size of a man 6 feet tall, weighing 170 pounds, but you never got that impression when one actually saw him."

Robert's family had no history of giantism. His father was of average size at 5 feet 10 inches, weighing 150 pounds. His mother was petite at 5 feet 4 inches, 120 pounds. Robert's birth weight was only 8 1/2 pounds, nearly normal by today's standards. At age one, he exceeded an average baby's length by 30 percent.

MacBryde described Robert as "symmetrically formed, having beautifully shaped hands and no features of acromegaly in face, hands, feet or otherwise. His genitalia were normal in size, and his (arm) span was slightly less than his height. He had blue eyes, straight coarse blond hair, normal hair on his head, in axillae and on pubis, but very little hair on face, chest, abdomen and forearms. The eyes seemed smaller than would be proportionate to the huge skull."

X-rays of Robert's skull showed an enlarged sella turcia, measuring about 2.5 cm by 2.5 cm deep, apparently expanded by a pituitary tumor. "Studies on the Metabolism Ward at Barnes Hospital showed that he had a moderate iron-deficiency type of anemia and some calcium deficiency, with poorly calcified bones," MacBryde said. "He had disturbed sensation in the lower legs and feet, with loss of touch, pain and temperate sensibility. At about age 18 the joints of his knees, ankles and feet began to show compression deformities because of his immense weight and fragile bones. He developed severe flat feet. His bone and joint troubles interfered with walking, so for the last two or three years of his life he had to use one or two canes."

"During his most rapid growth period, when he was 15 to 17 years old, he required 7,500 calories daily. During that last two years when he was still growing, but not at such a phenomenal rate, he needed about 4,500 calories per day. We felt that his osteam lacia, anemia, bone collapse and neuropathy were due to nutritional inadequacies and treated him with a diet and vitamin and iron supplements. He improved, and we thought he would live for many years. He was still growing. In the last two years of his life, he still continued to gain about 2 1/2 inches of height per year."

MacBryde described Robert Wadlow as intelligent and pleasant, always a cooperative young man.

"His I.Q. was 124 and 116 on a repeated tests at intervals of years," MacBryde said. "He was a good student in high school and had one year at Shurtleff College in Alton. He was a formidable basketball center until ruled out of the league."

MacBryde said the group of doctors at Barnes were unable to secure permission for an autopsy after Robert's death because of the Wadlow family dispute with the Barnes Hospital colleague.

A cast of Wadlow's hand was made when he was 18. Dr. MacBryde said it was 11-3/8 inches from wrist line to tip of middle finger. The last measurement of the hand at age 22 years, 4 3/4 months from the previous measurement was 12-3/4 inches. A man 6-feet tall has a hand about 7-3/4 inches long. Wadlow's last shoe was a size 37 and 18-1/2 inches long. An average 6-foot man wears a size 10-1/2 shoe and 12-1/4 inches long. Dr. Louis H. Behrens of Barnes Hospital made a careful study of Robert's growth since he was a mere 7-footer.

Unlike most other giants, Robert's growth began at birth, Dr. Behrens said. When he was 13, his physical strength increased markedly. Robert played basketball so well that his team did not lose a game, and he once took a 13-mile hike without fatigue. Except for his extraordinary size, Robert was a normal boy for his age, doing well in classes both in high school and in his freshman year at Shurtleff College in Alton. Dr. Behrens called Robert "studious and mentally capable."

Robert's problems came from his feet. In 1930, 1931, two times in 1932 and again in 1935 he entered Barnes Hospital with infections or broken bones in his feet. He had little sensation in his feet and consequently did not feel a wrinkle in his sock or a pebble in his shoe until a blister was formed.

Dr. Behrens agreed that Robert's phenomenal growth was due to the abnormal activity of the pituitary gland. In normal-sized humans, the gland is lodged in a small pocket of bone near the base of the brain and is small. It is known that in some cases of giantism the pituitary gland has been as large as a hen's egg.

Dr. Behrens said Robert Wadlow was doubtless the tallest human giant. "We hear of others, but the facts about them have not been corroborated."

John F. Carroll of Buffalo, N.Y., was the next tallest person in medical history at 8 feet 7-3/4 inches. Carroll died in 1969 at age 37.

Charles Byme, whose body was recovered from the seas, was reputed to be 8 feet 4 inches, but actually was only 7 feet 7. John Turner, often referred to as 8 feet 4, was only 7 feet 7. Cornelius Magrath, whose skeleton is in Dublin, Ireland, was reported to be 8 feet 6 but was only 7 fect 2-1/4 inches.

After Carroll would be John William Rogan, of Gallatin, Tenn., at 8 feet 6 inches. Dan Koehler, born in 1926, of Chicago, was 8 feet 2 inches.

Harold Wadlow Jr. believed that Robert would forever remain the world's tallest man. "They can control growth now with modern medicine," he said. "If someone gets to be that tall, they will have to be from another country other than here."

The question is why is everyone so fascinated with tall people? Harold thought he had the answer. "I'm fascinated by it," he said. "There used to be one fellow in Chicago who was a tall guy. He was almost 8 feet tall. He worked for a meat packing company. Way back then, kids were small. I guess we are all fascinated.

"People are still interested in all the facts about Robert. I don't think they will feel any different than we do in the future. The generation that grew up with Robert was before TV; this was all they had. He was an oddity that people talked about. People saw him. He was something nobody else was."

Harold said when he traveled throughout the country, he occasionally stopped at a hotel and registered under the name Wadlow. Often a desk clerk will ask, "You're from Alton, Illinois. Isn't Alton, Illinois, the home of Robert Wadlow, the world's tallest man?"

Harold said the clerk usually looked back at his name and say, "Your name is Wadlow. Are you related?" Typically Harold smiled back and told them the family story.

"It's amazing how Robert's name spread," Harold Jr. said. "The older people, not the younger crowd, remember. People have a lot of memories of him. It was a shame he died at 22. He was too young to die. I do want younger people to remember him, too."

Chapter 19

Alton's Favorite Son

Telegraph reporter Ande Yakstis spent much of his 40-year career writing stories and sharing memories about Robert Wadlow. Yakstis retired from the newspaper in November 2001, but even today when he travels throughout the area someone often asks him about the "Gentle Giant."

Yakstis first came into contact with Robert when he was 6 years old in 1939 at the Bethalto Homecoming. Hundreds cheered Robert that August day in a personal appearance at the homecoming. Yakstis has helped preserve the memories the public has today of the Alton man. Yakstis describes Wadlow as an "American legend" for his height and gentle personality.

"He was a giant but an ordinary person who loved to go to Downtown Alton shopping and to have fun with his friends, whether it was being a Boy Scout, church activities or being a DeMolay," Yakstis said. "He was an ordinary American. He loved his country and flag. He would go with his family each year to Alton's annual Memorial Day Parade, which is the oldest in the United States. He would admire the World War I veterans pass by. "Robert represented what was good about America. He was a real patriot. Robert loved birthday parties and even had a lemonade stand along Brown Street in Alton on hot summer days."

Childhood friend June Pitts Bassford feels Robert will be remembered as a "good, kindly, life-loving friend who was beloved by everyone who knew him. Now he belongs to the world," she said.

Another childhood friend, Lee Duncan, often stops by the Wadlow Statue and is amazed at the attention Robert garners today on College Avenue.

"To me, and to the guys who hung out in Pie Town, in many ways, Robert was no big deal," Duncan said. "He was our friend and we were used to him."

Robert Landiss is hopeful Alton never lets Robert Wadlow's memory escape the community. "Because of the type of person he was, he was a friendly person to everybody, I hope we always remember him here," he said. "To us he was just another person, not a freak. The only difference between us and him is he was twice as big as us."

Pat Turk today lives in Robert's last home at 2416 Sanford Ave. in Alton. The Wadlow family never owned the house but rented from Turk's mother, Clara Telkamp. Pat and her husband, Leo, moved into the house in 1970 after inheriting it.

Sightseers constantly drive by on tours of Alton to see where Robert last resided. Occasionally, the historical society brings people over to see the Sanford Avenue residence. Leo Turk knew Robert. He told stories through the years of setting up two folding chairs in the back of the Uptown Theater for Robert when he attended the movies. An usher would always be stationed at the back of the theater with Robert to make sure children didn't trip over him.

The Sanford Avenue dwelling only had 9-foot ceilings, which made it difficult for Robert to navigate through the house. Pat Turk's favorite photo is with Harold Jr. peeking around the corner of the front entrance of the house with Robert.

Alton Mayor Don Sandidge first learned about Robert Wadlow as a little boy. Robert has been a "symbol of Alton" to Sandidge since his childhood.

"My father, Tom Sandidge, and Robert went to school at the same time," Don Sandidge said. "My father kept my brother and I informed about Robert. We get inquiries today about Robert from all over the world. There is always someone visiting his statue. Robert is really a hot topic on the Internet today. Robert is something positive for the city to hang its hat on."

Greg Gelzinnis, owner of Bluff City Tours in Alton, continually takes people by the Wadlow statue and tells the story of the city's giant. Gelzinnis, too, sees Wadlow as a hero for Alton residents.

"Robert Wadlow was somebody everybody can relate to, either seniors or children," Gelzinnis said. "He was a role model by being a positive person and willing to be as normal as he could. He wanted to have a sled and have a lemonade stand. He was like you and me and wanted to be plain Robert."

On Gelzinnis' Alton tours, he always makes the Wadlow Statue his first stop. "I'd say on tours, five of 30 people saw him on a tour in their hometown or have a story from a mother, father, aunt or uncle," he said. "It's been fun over the years to hear those people's stories. The statue helped make people aware of him. I guess I have taken nearly 10,000 to 25,000 people to see his statue."

Crown Optical at 406 Broadway in Alton added a statue of Robert Wadlow in February 1995 that constantly draws attention from customers and passers-by. The statue was created in 1991 by Pat Schuchard, a full-time professor and head of the art program at Washington University in St. Louis.

The Crown Optical statue head and hands are made of clay and are slightly smaller than Robert's. The face does not look like Robert but supposedly is more of a facsimile, not a portrait. The hands and feet are made out of clay, a symbol of his sense of vulncrability, Schuchard said after unveiling the statue.

"Many people who go to the Alton Marina also come on over here to see the statue," Alton Crown Optical manager Barb Garis, now deceased, said. "We do have information people can read about it. It creates an atmosphere that was part of Downtown Alton. We just wanted to do something to be part of his life. He was such a great man and a gentle giant."

Scott Nuedecker, president of the Upper Alton Business Association, grew up as a DeMolay visiting the Masonic Temple in Upper Alton. Scott sat in the Wadlow Chair at the Masonic Temple as a youngster. The memory of that trip had such a lasting impact on Neudecker that as an adult he decided to start a drive to erect a replica near the Wadlow Statue.

On Oct. 20, 2002, the Wadlow Chair was dedicated next to the statue. Nearly $80,000 was raised, primarily through selling bricks and blocks.

"It is a great enhancement to the statue site," Neudecker said. "There is a lot of interest in Robert Wadlow. This will help people who are trying to visualize what it would have been like being his size. Everything else in the world at his time was built for someone about 6-feet tall."

The Upper Alton Business Association led Alton area civic groups in raising enough money to position the chair near the Wadlow Statue. The Alton-Godfrey Rotary Club was another large contributor in the fund drive.

Gene Crivello of Alton thinks having a replica of Robert's chair next to the statue was a good idea. "People can sit in the chair and have pictures taken," he said. "Robert Wadlow is something Alton should be very proud of. We in Alton have a citizen, born right here, who was the tallest man to ever live on the face of the earth and was just a wonderful, caring young man."

Robert's death in 1940 was a sudden blow to the people of Alton, Crivello said.

"Robert got heavier as he got older and the braces on his legs wore a blister on his heel," Crivello said. "Imagine carrying 500 pounds with a 42 shoe. If he had continued to live, I think he would have ended up in a wheelchair and possibly been bedridden eventually."

A movement has begun to preserve the small house where Robert was born at 1421 Monroe St. in Alton. Charlene Gill, president emeritus of the Alton Museum of History & Art, believes it is important to preserve the home and Wadlow's first memories. In late 2001, the house was moved to SIUE Dental School campus. The Alton Museum signed a 99-year lease with the SIUE Board. The Wadlow birth home is situated northwest of the Wadlow Statue and a brick path will wind its way to the four-room house that will be furnished by David Culp, vice president of the Alton Museum. A living room, dining room, kitchen and bathroom will be furnished as it might have been on Feb. 22, 1918 — the day Robert Pershing Wadlow was born there.

Alton Township Supervisor Don Huber thinks Robert Wadlow personifies the calm, Midwestern attitude in the quaint river city. He said Robert seemed to accept what happened to him and make the best of his situation.

"He personifies what is good about Alton to the rest of the nation and world," Huber said. "Robert was able to live a normal life in spite of his awful disability. He handled all the insults and insensitivity of people with grace and dignity. We need to be indebted to him for remaining gentle and polite even when his height thrust him into the limelight.

"All the people I know who grew up with him say he remained a nice guy and a gentle guy no matter what people said. I think his gentle part is even more important than him being a giant. Robert Wadlow is Alton's favorite son."

Chapter 20

Family Reunion

On a warm August day in 2000, Harold Wadlow Jr. eased his beige 1993 four-door Ford Escort to the side of the road on College Avenue directly across the street from the lifelike bronze statue of his brother. As usual, several people had congregated at the statue.

Harold tried to remain incognito that day. Two nuns were giving about 15 people a tour. Harold sat quietly in his car but yearned to go out and tell them the whole Robert Wadlow story. But the final surviving child of Harold Sr. and Addie Wadlow decided to remain in his car to watch the two nuns and tour group for 10 or 15 minutes.

Harold Jr. wanted to stay out of the limelight after watching his brother, Robert, on center stage and his father, Harold Sr., wrestle in the Alton political arena as an alderman and mayor.

"I got married and moved to St. Louis to begin with," Harold Jr. said. "When Mother and Dad were still living, I was over here every other weekend. It was surprising when we later lived in Tennessee and Alabama and when people found out what my name was, they asked about Robert. I was a quiet person. There was always Robert, after that my father was mayor and in politics. I preferred to stay in the background and just be quiet and observe."

Harold Jr. had to overcome his shyness when he worked with the Veteran's Administration office in St. Louis. He was a section chief, which required considerable public speaking. After a while, he said he got used to talking in front of groups and crowds. He retreated from interviews during his final years because of a negative experience with a British television taping.

"We had one interview for five hours," he said. "When it came on television I was on for a quick flip and was off. That was one of my breaking points in 1999."

Harold Jr. often made the trip to the Wadlow Statue to watch people measuring and comparing themselves against his gigantic brother. In fact, trips to the Robert Wadlow Statue felt like a trek home.

"There is a crowd at Robert's statue every time I drive down the street," he said. "People are still interested in him 60 years after his death. To me, I've lived with it all my life. I'm used to it."

Tourists come to Alton from around the world to visit the statue and the Alton Museum of History & Art to see a detailed display about the world's tallest man. "Robert put Alton on the map," Harold Jr. proclaims.

"Robert always treated me like I was a king," he said. "I was his baby brother. He didn't want me to have to put up with all the stuff that he did. I can't imagine what it was like for him, but I think it was like being a soldier in a war and returning home. People opened doors for him. He was very gentle, especially with me. My memories of him will always be the best."

Often, Harold Jr. reflected on what Robert could have accomplished if he had lived past 22.

"He was quiet and gentle," Harold Jr. said. "Robert loved people. He was too young to die. I think there is a lot more he could have done with his life ahead."

Harold Jr. felt Robert's most remarkable achievement was

being able to handle all the attention and remaining a kind and gentle character. Robert remained kind and gentle despite never having peace and quiet.

"He couldn't even go out of the house," Harold Jr. said. "He couldn't just go to the store like we do or get an ice cream cone at a drugstore soda fountain. He couldn't go anywhere without people staring. There was no television back then; he was really an oddity. He couldn't go out without people looking."

Harold Jr. was uncertain if he thought Robert believed he wouldn't see old age. He said Robert's longevity was never discussed in the family before his death.

"People like Robert don't usually live to be old with problems like he had. I don't think he or my family had any idea of how long he would live."

When Harold Jr. traveled or did things with Robert, the thing he remembers most is everyone looking and staring. "I was used to it. It was everywhere we went," he said. "I was 8 when he died. When you're used to that, you think nothing of people looking."

Robert was quoted as saying that when people stared or made fun of him, he knew they couldn't help it. "I've gotten used to being stared at," Robert once told an interviewer in the late 1930s. "I thought it over a long time ago and told myself to ignore them. The worst thing you can say about them is that they are thoughtless."

The Rev. William Fester, Main Street Methodist Church pastor, performed the funeral for Addie Wadlow in late December 1980 at Smith Funeral Home in Alton. Fester remembers the Wadlows as being very nice people.

"All of them went to church here," Fester said of the Wadlow family. "Mr. Wadlow was heavily involved in politics, serving as a mayor for one term and as an alderman. When I used to visit Addie in her home, she would always seem to revert to talking about Robert. Addie would always say, 'He was a good boy.' The Wadlow family tried to keep people from making him

149

into a freak. She said she tried to make sure Robert had as normal a life as possible. Robert's mother and family dearly loved him as their child."

Fester thinks many people forgot in Robert's highly publicized life that he was Harold Sr. and Addie Wadlow's son, and not just the world's tallest man. Thousands of visitors have paid tribute to the world's tallest man's grave through time. The family always felt secure after the vault and concrete was placed that Robert would be safe in the cemetery.

When Harold Jr. visited Shop 'N Save in Alton, he often drove past the Wadlow family plot in Upper Alton Cemetery.

"I can't help but think about things a lot when I come out here," he said during the summer of 2000. "I have a lot of memories of my wife, Robert, my mother and father and sisters."

Harold Jr. grew up speaking publicly about his famous big brother. It helped working for the Veterans Administration in St. Louis and delivering speeches constantly on his job.

"I enjoyed talking about Robert," Harold Jr. said. "It made me a private person in some ways I think, growing up the way I did with Robert in the spotlight."

Harold said that every once in a while in deep sleep Robert slipped into his dreams. It's almost like Robert was still here with Harold Jr. 60 years after he was laid to rest on that hot, July day.

During the summer of 2000, Harold Jr. didn't feel that he had a lot of time left on earth after suffering several small strokes and experiencing various health problems. He thought then it was time to tell his side of Robert's story and record the memories of the other elderly Alton area townspeople.

"I'm gradually getting weaker," he said at the time. "It's probably good we are getting these things done now."

Harold Jr. said Robert gave him everything he could have possibly wanted in a big brother. Robert became worldly from his travels and knew a lot.

"Robert met senators, governors and a lot of important people," Harold Jr. said. "Robert was of above average intelligence. His handicap was trying to get around. He just wasn't mobile at all. He liked people. He tried to cooperate with people as much as he could. He worked with the church, Boy Scouts and was a member of the Masons. Betty and I were like Robert; Helen and Eugene were alike. My fondest memory of him is all the attention he gave me."

Barbara Ellen Upchurch, Robert Wadlow's niece, said the questions have been unending about him.

"I have a young son who was named Robert in honor of my uncle and to express my pride for my family," Upchurch said. "The family always protected Robert's memory as fervently when I was growing up as they did while he was alive. We were just naturally following in Grandpa's footsteps; I think it was almost instinctive. I suppose that was because we lived it all our lives and knew how important it was to our grandparents... they were devoted to all their children, but Robert was the one who needed protecting, and the family all did this together with great love and strength as a unit."

Addie was found dead at her home on Oscar Avenue in Alton on Dec. 25, 1980. Robert's brother, Eugene H. Wadlow, died in 1959 at 37 of a heart attack, and sister Helen I. Wilson died Feb. 4, 1989, at age 78. Robert's other sister, Betty Brada, died in 1980 at 66. Betty's son, Robert Brada, is buried next to her in the Wadlow family plot. Harold Jr.'s wife, Kimma, is also buried with the rest of the family. She died at age 48 in 1996.

The Wadlow family plot is found in an area in Oakwood Cemetery in Upper Alton. Robert Wadlow's grave stands above the others engraved with "At Rest, Robert Wadlow, Feb. 22, 1918-July 1940." Harold Sr. and Addie Wadlow purchased 22 lots in the cemetery for their family when Robert died.

Robert's grave is flanked by his mother and father's graves and those of his two sisters, brother and sister-in-law. Harold Sr. died Sept. 26, 1969, collapsing on the Alton Municipal Golf Course after a heart attack. Golfing partners attempted to revive him with mouth-to-mouth resuscitation and artificial respiration, but to no avail. Ironically years later the city of Alton renamed municipal golf course after its favorite son Robert Wadlow.

"My wife, Kimma, died suddenly in the middle of the night," Harold Jr. said. "We don't know what happened. I went to sleep in my recliner. When I went in the bedroom the next morning, she was lying there dead."

Kim Tyler, one of Harold Jr.'s daughters, said her father was very proud of the Wadlow family history and had a special relationship with Robert.

Harold Jr.'s other daughter, Lisa Wadlow, said her lasting memory of her father was that "he loved me and loved my family."

"He was always really concerned that we were happy, healthy and that things were going well in our lives," Lisa Wadlow said.

Harold Jr. believed having a big brother so loving and caring helped him instill the same principles in his two daughters, Kim and Lisa.

"I didn't care what they did with their lives; I just wanted them to be happy and healthy," Harold Jr. said. "Those two things were most important to me."

Tyler said she used to be asked to talk about her famous uncle, Robert, while attending Fox High in Arnold, Mo.

"We were very proud of Uncle Robert," she said. "When we were young, we didn't know anything except the basic facts about him. I know Dad and Robert were really close and that Robert was really fond of my dad."

Tyler said her family didn't talk about Robert incessantly. "It was just a part of our lives," Tyler said. "We didn't see it as unusual. Sometimes people would talk about Uncle Robert and it would be really nice and we were proud. I am kind of shy and didn't like a lot of attention."

Lisa Wadlow said it was hard for her family to comprehend

Robert's fame.

"He was my Uncle Robert; he was just a part of my family," she said. "Once in a while people find out my last name is Wadlow and ask if I am related. I just tell them he was my uncle. It's hard to believe that for most people it is such a big deal. He was just my uncle, and he was the tallest recorded person in history. I'm more private about everything than my dad. I wish there wasn't as much attention about Robert, although I understand people's curiosity."

"Robert wasn't mentioned more than anyone else in my family," she said. "I do know my dad was his favorite sibling. There was a special relationship between the two of them."

Harold Jr. said during the summer of 2000 that it was often lonely being the only remaining family member of Harold Sr. and Addie Wadlow.

"I lost my wife, mother, father, two brothers, two sisters, aunts, uncles," Harold Jr. said. "It's difficult sometimes being the last surviving member of the immediate Wadlow family."

Asked which photo of him and Robert was his favorite, Harold Jr. responded, "The Leland Heppner photo of me peeking around the corner with Robert. That was me, 'Mr. Mischief.'"

Harold Jr. appeared to be the closest to Robert of all his siblings. Through the years, he retained those precious memories. "It's all up here," he said, pointing at his temple. "Robert and I were a lot alike. He loved me as his little brother. We were both quiet and gentle."

In his last public interview only a few weeks before his death, Harold Jr. sighed and looked to the heavens while sitting near Robert's grave at Upper Alton Cemetery.

"I hope I get to see him in heaven some day," Harold Jr. said. "If I do, I'd love to tell him how things turned out for me and my family. I'll tell him about my life and my kids, Lisa and Kim. I would love to tell him how people would ask my girls about him when they were in school and when they talked about him. I think he would be proud."

At 5:19 p.m. on Dec. 31, 2000, Harold Jr. died at Alton Memorial Hospital. On the afternoon of Jan. 5, 2001, he was laid to rest in Upper Alton Cemetery next to his brother, Robert, on a beautiful, winter day. Snow had drifted around the tombstones in the cemetery on Oakwood Road in Alton. The two brothers were finally reunited after being apart for more than 60 years.

One of Harold Jr.'s last statements was: "I was the apple of his eye. What he didn't know was he was the apple of mine."

Boy Giant

Alton, Illinois
Key Historical Facts

Alton, Ill., with a population of 31,000, is a historic community on the Mississippi River, about 30 miles north of St. Louis.

The area immediately north and west of the city is famed for its scenic bluffs. Alton was the site of the debate between U.S. Senate candidates Abraham Lincoln and Stephen A. Douglas in 1858 that drew thousands to the area. Today, Lincoln-Douglas Square in Downtown Alton features lifelike statues of the two political "giants" of their day.

Alton began as a steamboat town and has an abundance of Mississippi River heritage. Explorers Meriwether Lewis and William Clark made their camp during the winter of 1803-1804 in Wood River, Ill., just outside Alton, before starting their historic journey to the west by paddling across the Mississippi to its confluence with the Missouri River.

The Piasa Bird legend remains in Alton. In memory of a young brave who was killed trying to slay the Piasa Bird near Alton, several pictures of the bird were painted on the area's bluffs. During the 1990s, a large metal sculpture of the bird was removed from a quarry site just outside Alton. Today, the Piasa Bird has been repainted on the rock face of the bluffs, about two miles west of Alton. The myth surrounding the Piasa Bird continues to be passed from generation to generation.

During the Civil War, thousands of Confederate prisoners of war were held at a prison in Alton, and thousands of them died there, mainly from yellow fever. Before and during the war, Alton was one of the main depots of three Illinois Underground Railroad routes. The free lands of Alton were separated from St. Louis, one of the largest slave areas north of New Orleans, only by the Mississippi River. Quickly, it became a prime location sought by slaves in their quest for freedom.

On Nov. 15, 1837, Alton suffered a devastating blow when Elijah P. Lovejoy, an abolitionist newspaper editor, was murdered by a pro-slavery mob. Lovejoy was protecting his Alton Observer presses. He defended the presses along the river in Alton at Gilman's Warehouse, where he was shot. The presses were hauled to the nearby Mississippi River and destroyed. For years after, Alton was scorned by some Americans because of the Lovejoy incident. Alton was labeled as a "racist," and many businesses and industries settled in more tolerant areas.

Alton's problems with racism continued through the 1960s when native James Earl Ray was convicted of murdering civil rights activist Dr. Martin Luther King Jr. on April 4, 1968, in Memphis, Tenn. Ray was born March 10, 1928, at 1021 W. Ninth St. in Alton.

The Alton area was also the scene of the much-publicized Paula Sims murder case. Sims was convicted in 1990 of murdering her 6-week-old daughter, Heather, in a warm bath and killing 13-day-old Loralei the same way in 1986 when the family lived in Jersey County. Sims' story was the basis for "Precious Victims," a best-selling book written by former Madison County State's Attorney Don Weber and former St. Louis Post-Dispatch reporter Charles Bosworth Jr., and later a two-hour television movie.

The Great River Road outside Alton was named to the National Scenic Byway list in Washington, D.C., in 1998. Only about 20 highways are on the National Scenic Byway group.

The author Dan Brannan is executive editor of the Telegraph, In Alton, IL. Brannan resides in Alton with his wife, Victoria, and daughters, Savannah, and Sierra.

BOY GIANT contains family memories, area memories and chronicles the life of Robert Wadlow, including his U.S. tours, life in Alton as a Boy Scout, Mason, involvement with the United Methodist Church, his medical history, death and funeral. It also tells the story behind the Alton Museum, the Wadlow Statue effort, the Wadlow Chair and Wadlow House renovation.

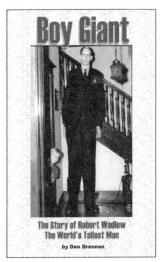

Boy Giant

The Story of Robert Wadlow
The World's Tallest Man
by Dan Brannan

To order copies send a check or money order to:

Alton Museum of History and Art, Inc.
2809 College Ave.,
Alton, IL 62002
or call 618-462-2763

Name:_____

Signature of Buyer_____

Address:_____

City:_____ State:_____ Zip:_____

The book is $19.95, plus $1.42 tax and $4 shipping and handling. For quantity discounts, call 618-462-2763.

CUSTOMER RECEIPT

Name:_____

Signature of Buyer_____

Address:_____

City:_____ State:_____ Zip:_____

Editor's Note: Anyone who would like to submit a written account or photograph involving Robert Wadlow to be displayed at the Alton Museum, please send to:
Dan Brannan, 2611 Dennis Dr., Alton, IL 62002

Also by Dan Brannan....

"Life to The Fullest: Stories of People Coping With Diabetes"

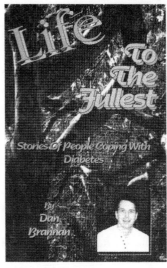

A practical guide to life for those with diabetes and their families, written by a person with diabetes, who knows what it's like to live with the disease day to day.

To order your copy, just send a check or money order for $12.95 plus 91 cents tax and $4 shipping and handling (per copy) to:

Dan Brannan
2611 Dennis Dr.
Alton, IL 62002

Name:_____

Address:_____

City, State, Zip Code:_____

No. of Copies:_____Amount Enclosed:_____

For Quantity Discounts, Call: 618-465-9275